Rapid Reference Review in Orthopedic Trauma

Pivotal Papers Revealed

T0198145

Rapid Reference Review in Orthopedic Trauma

Pivotal Papers Revealed

David J. Hak, MD, MBA, FACS

Professor
Orthopedic Surgery, Denver Health
University of Colorado
Denver, Colorado

SLACK
INCORPORATED

www.Healio.com/books

ISBN: 978-1-61711-048-1

Copyright © 2013 by SLACK Incorporated

David J. Hak has no financial or proprietary interest in the materials presented herein.

Published by: SLACK Incorporated
                     6900 Grove Road
                     Thorofare, NJ 08086 USA
                     Telephone: 856-848-1000
                     Fax: 856-848-6091
                     www.Healio.com/books

Contact SLACK Incorporated for more information about other books in this field or about the availability of our books from distributors outside the United States.

Library of Congress Cataloging-in-Publication Data

Rapid reference review in orthopedic trauma : pivotal papers revealed / David J. Hak.
    p. ; cm.
Includes bibliographical references and index.
ISBN 978-1-61711-048-1 (alk. paper)
[DNLM: 1. Fractures, Bone--Meta-Analysis. 2. Clinical Trials as Topic--Meta-Analysis. 3. Cohort Studies--Meta-Analysis. 4. Dislocations--Meta-Analysis. 5. Orthopedics--methods--Meta-Analysis. 6. Research Design--Meta-Analysis. WE 175]
    RD684
    617.4'7044--dc23
                        2013006482

Printed in the United States of America.

Last digit is print number: 10 9 8 7 6 5 4 3 2 1

Dedication

For Kimberly and Hailey, the pivotal people in my life.

Contents

About the Author

David J. Hak, MD, MBA, FACS graduated from the University of Michigan and received his medical degree from Ohio State University. His postdoctoral training included an orthopedic residency at the University of California at Los Angeles and an orthopedic trauma fellowship at the University of California at Davis. He received his MBA in health care administration from Auburn University. He has been on the faculty of the University of Michigan, the University of California at Davis, and the University of Colorado. Dr. Hak is a fellow of the American Academy of Orthopaedic Surgeons and the American College of Surgeons. He serves in various leadership roles in the Orthopaedic Trauma Association and the International Society for Fracture Repair.

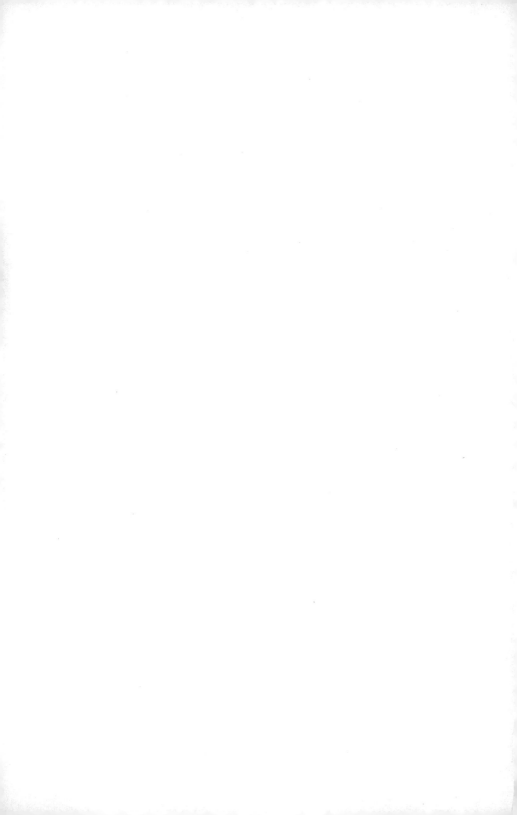

Introduction

Attempting to select "pivotal" papers is undoubtedly an impossible task that, by necessity, leaves out hundreds of equally important, or even more important, articles. In order to achieve a concise list of pivotal papers, the following criteria have been considered:

- ▶ Prospective, randomized clinical studies (Level I evidence)
- ▶ Large prospective clinical cohort studies
- ▶ Meta-analyses of published series
- ▶ Articles that are commonly cited, either in the literature or during teaching conferences
- ▶ Top-cited articles published in the *Journal of Orthopaedic Trauma*, 1987 to 2007
- ▶ Articles recommended by the Orthopaedic Trauma Association Evidence-Based Medicine Project Team in 2007
- ▶ When possible, I have focused on clinical studies, rather than anatomic or biomechanical studies

In addition, there is a wide variability in the number of potential pivotal papers to select from in different anatomic areas. Therefore, some chapters may have articles that you may consider of relatively low importance, while other chapters may omit well-designed prospective randomized clinical trials. There is also wide variation in the rigor of individual studies because they span many decades during which research and publication standards have changed.

The exclusion of any article from this text should not lead the reader to minimize its worth. Invariably, the authors of these other articles are well justified in feeling slighted and can rightfully question why their article was not included. As already mentioned, any attempt to select pivotal articles is an impossible task given the wide range of important and worthwhile papers.

As the medical information expands at an exponential pace, the ability to quickly identify relevant articles using PubMed becomes increasingly difficult. It is my hope that readers will find this text useful in their education and practice. Orthopedic trainees may be able to quickly review several articles in preparation for a morning conference presentation of patients with a specific fracture, while practicing surgeons may be able to advise patients on the relative benefits of one treatment over another.

In addition to pivotal papers, I have included selected review articles for each chapter. Additional review material can also be found in the American

Academy of Orthopaedic Surgeons Instructional Course Lectures and in the Cochrane Reviews.

We are all indebted to the hard work of the authors of articles reviewed in this text, for their efforts and knowledge are what has helped us all advance the care of our patients. Any errors and omissions in the material presented are my responsibility, not the original authors.

Finally, while I have attempted to abstract the key findings from each paper, I would encourage you to read the complete paper for a thorough understanding of the methods and findings. Like any review book, these annotated references are intended to serve as a guide and not as a replacement for the original work. The reader may also notice differences in numbers reported in this text with those in the papers abstracts. Abstracts often refer to the total number of patients eligible for study and, for clarity, I have usually tried to provide the numbers used in the final data analysis.

The following standard abbreviations/notations are used in the text:

▶ AP = anteroposterior

▶ CT = computed tomography

▶ DVT = deep vein thrombosis

▶ IM = intramedullary

▶ IV = intravenous

▶ L = liter

▶ MRI = magnetic resonance imaging

▶ ORIF = open reduction and internal fixation

▶ OTA = Orthopaedic Trauma Association

▶ Preop = preoperative

▶ Postop = postoperative

▶ SF-36 = Short Form-36

▶ SF-12 = Short Form-12

▶ ROM = range of motion

▶ VAS = Visual Analog Scale

▶ Where a set of two numbers appears in parentheses, this indicates the range of values. For example: average age 38 years (22 to 68 years)

David J. Hak, MD, MBA, FACS

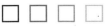

Calcaneus Fractures

chapter 1

CLASSIC ARTICLE

Authors: Sanders R, Fortin P, DiPasquale T, Walling A.

Title: Operative treatment in 120 displaced intraarticular calcaneal fractures. Results using a prognostic computed tomography scan classification.

Journal Information: *Clin Orthop Relat Res.* 1993;290:87–95.

▸ This classic article defines the Sanders Classification for calcaneus fractures.

▸ Authors developed a classification system based on the degree of intra-articular posterior facet injury on standardized coronal and transverse CT scans (Sanders Classification)

  ▷ Type I: nondisplaced (all treated nonoperatively)

  ▷ Type II: 2-part or split fractures

  ▷ Type III: 3-part or split-depression fractures

  ▷ Type IV: 4-part or highly comminuted articular fractures

Study Design: Retrospective Review

▸ 132 displaced calcaneus fractures treated with ORIF.

▸ 120 had minimum 1-year follow-up

  ▷ Average follow-up: 29 months (12 to 56 months)

Hak DJ.
*Rapid Reference Review in Orthopedic Trauma:
Pivotal Papers Revealed (pp 1-15).*
© 2013 SLACK Incorporated.

- Outcome measurements
  - ▷ Maryland Foot Score (MFS)
  - ▷ Postop CT scans

Results

- Restoration of heel height (98%), width (110%), and length (100%) to virtually normal in all cases, regardless of preop displacement.
- Anatomic articular reduction in 86% of type II fractures, 60% of type III, and 0% of type IV.
- Excellent or good clinical results in 73% of type II fractures, 70% of type III, and 9% of type IV.

Conclusions

- The authors noted a distinct learning curve with improved clinical results for type II and III fractures in later years of their surgical experience.
- Although anatomic articular reduction is necessary for a good result, it did not guarantee a good result.
- Patients with type IV fractures can expect inferior operative results irrespective of the surgeon's experience, and the authors recommended that consideration should be given to primary arthrodesis.

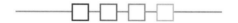

FEATURED ARTICLE

Authors: Buckley R, Tough S, McCormack R, et al.

Title: Operative compared with nonoperative treatment of displaced intra-articular calcaneal fractures: a prospective, randomized, controlled multicenter trial.

Journal Information: *J Bone Joint Surg Am.* 2002;84-A(10): 1733–1744.

Study Design: Prospective, Multicenter, Randomized Study

▸ 424 patients with 471 displaced intra-articular calcaneal fractures treated at 4 trauma centers were randomized to operative or nonoperative care.

▸ Final study population consisted of 309 patients (161 operative, 148 nonoperative) with a minimum 2-year follow-up.

▸ Inclusion criteria: Age 15 to 68, intra-articular calcaneal fracture displaced > 2 mm from anatomic position as demonstrated by axial and coronal CT scanning of the posterior facet.

▸ Exclusion criteria: Medical contraindications to surgery, previous calcaneal abnormality (an infection or a tumor), previous calcaneal injury, coexistent foot injury, an extra-articular fracture, an open calcaneal fracture, an injury that had occurred more than 14 days before presentation, and head injury.

▸ Each surgeon was required to enroll and follow a minimum of 20 patients. Patients in this study were treated by 6 surgeons from 4 centers. One surgeon treated 73% of the patients.

▸ Operative treatment consisted of a standard protocol using a lateral approach and rigid internal fixation. Nonoperative treatment consisted of initial ice, elevation, and rest. After 6 weeks of nonweightbearing, all patients began a standardized regimen with full weightbearing.

▸ Patients were seen at 2 to 4, 6, 12, 26, and 52 weeks and at 2 years.

▸ Outcome measurements
  ▷ SF-36 at 1 and 2 years
  ▷ VAS at 1 and 2 years

Results

▸ Overall, when all patient data were combined, there was no significant difference in the outcomes between the operative and nonoperative groups.

▸ However, the outcomes of some specific subgroups that were not receiving Workers' Compensation were significantly better with ORIF.

▸ The non-Workers' Compensation patients treated with ORIF had significantly higher satisfaction scores compared to those treated nonoperatively ($P = .001$).

▸ Females treated with ORIF scored significantly higher on the SF-36 compared to those treated nonoperatively ($P = .015$).

▶ Patients who did better with operative treatment were females; patients who were not receiving Workers' Compensation; younger males; patients with a higher Böhler's angle; patients with a lighter workload; and those with a single, simple displaced intra-articular calcaneal fracture.

▶ Anatomic or near-anatomic reductions improved outcomes, while comminuted reductions or fractures without reduction produced poorer long-term outcomes.

▶ Nonoperative care more commonly led to late arthrodesis.

▶ The best patients to treat nonoperatively were those 50 years or older, males, those receiving Workers' Compensation, and those whose occupation involves a heavy workload.

▶ The results after a higher-energy fracture (a lower Böhler's angle and more comminution) were not as good as those after a low-energy injury.

Conclusions

▶ Without group stratification, the functional results after nonoperative care of displaced intra-articular calcaneal fractures were equivalent to those after operative care.

▶ When patients who were receiving Workers' Compensation were excluded from analysis, the outcomes were significantly better in some groups of surgically treated patients.

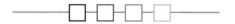

FEATURED ARTICLE

Authors: Potter MQ, Nunley JA.

Title: Long-term functional outcomes after operative treatment for intra-articular fractures of the calcaneus.

Journal Information: *J Bone Joint Surg Am.* 2009;91(8): 1854–1860.

Study Design: Retrospective Single-Center Review

▸ Intra-articular calcaneus fracture treated by fellowship-trained foot and ankle surgeons between 1989 and April 2003.

▸ 73 patients (81 fractures) provided follow-up functional questionnaire.

▸ Outcome measurements

▹ Adjusted American Orthopaedic Foot and Ankle Society (AOFAS) Ankle-Hindfoot Scale (subjective component only)

▹ Foot Function Index

▹ Calcaneal fracture scoring system

▸ Median of 12.8 years (5 to 18.5 years) after the injury.

Results

▸ Adjusted AOFAS Ankle-Hindfoot Scale: average 65.4.

▸ Foot Function Index: average 20.5.

▸ Calcaneal fracture scoring system: average 69.3.

▸ No significant difference in outcome between Workers' Compensation and non-Workers' Compensation.

▸ Patients whose injury was the result of a motor vehicle collision had significantly worse outcomes (Adjusted AOFAS and Foot Function Index) than those who sustained the injury in a fall.

▸ 13 (18%) patients had additional surgery on the injured foot or ankle: 7 hardware removal, 3 irrigation and débridement of a wound infection, 2 subtalar arthrodesis, and 1 tarsal tunnel release.

▸ Study limitations: retrospective nature, no nonoperative controls.

▸ Study strengths: long-term outcomes of a large cohort of calcaneus ORIF patients using validated outcome measures.

Conclusions

▸ The authors concluded that their long-term outcomes of calcaneal fracture ORIF were comparable to previously reported outcomes among smaller patient cohorts.

▸ They suggested additional investigation to determine why patients with fractures from a motor vehicle accident reported worse outcomes than patients with fractures from a fall.

Study Design: Retrospective Review

▸ Consecutive series of 69 patients with 75 displaced intra-articular calcaneal fractures who underwent subtalar arthrodesis for the treatment of painful post-traumatic subtalar arthritis.

▸ 34 patients (36 fractures) were initially managed with calcaneus ORIF and subsequently underwent in situ subtalar fusion at an average of 22.6 months later.

▸ 35 patients (39 fractures) were initially managed nonoperatively and developed a symptomatic painful malunion and subsequently underwent a subtalar distraction arthrodesis.

▸ The 2 groups were similar with respect to age, gender, injury mechanism, and smoking status.

▸ All complications were noted, and functional outcomes were assessed at a minimum of 48 months after fusion (average follow-up: 63 months).

Results

▸ 3 nonunions of the subtalar fusion requiring revision in each group.

▸ Patients initially treated with ORIF

▹ Fewer postop wound complications

▹ Significantly higher MFS (90.8 compared with 79.1; $P < .0001$)

▹ Significantly higher AOFAS Ankle-Hindfoot Scale (87.1 compared with 73.8; $P < .0001$)

Conclusions

▸ Authors concluded that initial ORIF restores calcaneal shape, alignment, and height, facilitating any future fusion procedure and establishing an opportunity to create a better long-term functional result.

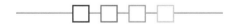

FEATURED ARTICLE

Authors: Folk JW, Starr AJ, Early JS.

Title: Early wound complications of operative treatment of calcaneus fractures: analysis of 190 fractures.

Journal Information: *J Orthop Trauma.* 1999;13(5):369–372.

Study Design: Retrospective Review

- 179 patients with 190 calcaneal fractures treated with ORIF.
- Average age: 35 years (17 to 77 years).
- Comorbidities
  - 9 diabetics
  - 111 cigarette smokers
  - 18 open fractures
- Average time from injury to surgery: 8 days (0 to 38 days).

Results

- 25% (48 patients) developed some form of wound complication.
- 21% (40 patients) required surgical treatment of the wound complication.
- Risk factors for wound complication
  - Diabetes (P = .02; relative risk 3.4)
  - Smoking (P = .03; relative risk 1.2)
  - Open fractures (P < .0001; relative risk 2.8)
  - The presence of more than one risk factor increased the relative risk of a wound complication requiring surgery

Conclusions

- Smoking, diabetes, and open fractures increase the risk of wound complication after calcaneus ORIF.
- The presence of more than one risk factor increases the likelihood of wound complications.

- Patients who have these risk factors should be counseled as to the possible complications that may arise after surgery.
- Consideration should be given to nonsurgical management in patients with multiple risk factors.

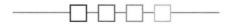

FEATURED ARTICLE
Authors: DeWall M, Henderson CE, McKinley TO, Phelps T, Dolan L, Marsh JL.
Title: Percutaneous reduction and fixation of displaced intra-articular calcaneus fractures.
Journal Information: *J Orthop Trauma*. 2010;24(8):466–472.

Study Design: Retrospective Cohort Study, Consecutive Series

- 125 intra-articular calcaneus fractures in 120 patients treated by 2 surgeons, one who performed primarily ORIF and one who performed primarily percutaneous treatment.
- Treatment was randomized by surgeon (although 9 crossover treatments in which the treating surgeon chose the other technique rather than the method they primarily performed) and time of presentation (when surgeon was on call)
  - ▷ 42 fractures treated by ORIF
    - » 32 joint depression
    - » 10 tongue type
    - » Sanders classification
      - ⟩ 19 type II
      - ⟩ 15 type III
      - ⟩ 1 type IV
      - ⟩ 7 unable to classify because CT scan was not available
  - ▷ 83 fractures treated by percutaneous reduction
    - » 61 joint depression
    - » 22 tongue type

> Sanders classification
> > 32 type II
> > 27 type III
> > 5 type IV
> > 19 unable to classify because CT scan was not available
- ORIF group had an extended lateral approach and fixation with plates and screws.
- Percutaneous group had small incisions with indirect fragment manipulation and fixation with screws alone.
- Outcome measurements
  - Clinical evaluation
  - Radiographic evaluation
- Average follow-up
  - 24.7 months (2 to 68 months) in ORIF group
  - 21.9 months (2 to 67 months) in percutaneous group

Results

- No difference in surgical improvement in Böhler's angle between the 2 treatment groups ($P = .31$)
  - Average: 22.4 degrees improvement in ORIF group
  - Average: 25.3 degrees improvement in percutaneous group
- No difference in loss of reduction at time of healing (minimum 4 months postop).
- Significantly higher deep infection rate in ORIF group ($P = .002$)
  - 14% (6/42) in ORIF group
  - 0% in percutaneous group
- Significantly higher minor wound complications in ORIF group ($P = .03$)
  - 21% (9/42) in ORIF group
  - 6% (5/83) in percutaneous group
- No difference in need for hardware removal
  - 12% (5/42) in ORIF group
  - 12% (10/83) in percutaneous group
- In 67 patients who had a minimum 2-year follow-up, there was no difference in the need for late subtalar fusion
  - 8% (2/26) in ORIF group
  - 7% (3/41) in percutaneous group

Conclusions

▸ Percutaneous reduction and fixation of calcaneus fractures minimizes the complications and both achieves and maintains extra-articular reduction (as measured by Böhler's angle) as well as ORIF.

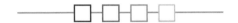

FEATURED ARTICLE

Authors: Tomesen T, Biert J, Frölke JP.

Title: Treatment of displaced intra-articular calcaneal fractures with closed reduction and percutaneous screw fixation.

Journal Information: *J Bone Joint Surg Am.* 2011;93(10):920–928.

Study Design: Retrospective Cohort Study

▸ 39 displaced intra-articular calcaneus fractures in 37 patients treated by closed reduction and percutaneous fixation with a minimum of 24-months follow-up.

▸ Average follow-up: 66 months (25 to 79 months).

▸ Outcome measurements
  ▷ AOFAS
  ▷ MFS
  ▷ SF-36
  ▷ Patient satisfaction (VAS)
  ▷ Radiographic evaluation

▸ Fracture type
  ▷ 12 tongue type
  ▷ 21 joint depression
  ▷ 5 comminuted
  ▷ 1 unclassified

▷ Sanders classification
  » 10 type II
  » 15 type III
  » 13 type IV
  » 1 unclassified

Results

▸ Complications
  ▷ 2 superficial wound infections
  ▷ 3 deep wound infections
  ▷ 2 patients underwent a subtalar arthrodesis because of persistent disabling pain due to subtalar arthritis
  ▷ 1 patient developed type I complex regional pain syndrome
  ▷ 4 patients had transient hypoesthesias or hyperesthesias
  ▷ 2 patients developed hammer-toe deformities
▸ Average outcome scores at final follow-up
  ▷ AOFAS: 84 points (26 to 100 points)
  ▷ MFS: 86 points (39 to 99 points)
  ▷ SF-36: 76 points (21 to 94 points)
  ▷ Satisfaction VAS: 7.9 points (4 to 10 points)
▸ Radiographic evaluation
  ▷ Average preop Böhler's angle: 3.4 degrees (–29 to 29 degrees)
  ▷ Average postop Böhler's angle: 21.8 degrees (5 to 43 degrees)
  ▷ Average Böhler's angle at final follow-up: 20.1 degrees (15 to 42 degrees)
▸ 78% of patients were able to wear normal shoes.
▸ 46% (17/37) of patients underwent hardware removal.
▸ 2 patients had undergone subtalar arthrodesis.

Conclusions

▸ The authors concluded that closed reduction and percutaneous reduction of intra-articular calcaneus fractures can produce a high degree of patient satisfaction in calcaneus fractures with small amounts of comminution (Sanders type II and type III), tongue-type fractures, and joint depression-type fractures provided that they have a sufficiently large tuberosity and sustentaculum fragment.

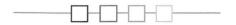

FEATURED ARTICLE
Authors: Potenza V, Caterini R, Farsetti P, Bisicchia S, Ippolito E.
Title: Primary subtalar arthrodesis for the treatment of comminuted intra-articular calcaneal fractures.
Journal Information: *Injury.* 2010;41(7):702–706.

Study Design: Retrospective Cohort Study

▶ 7 markedly comminuted intra-articular calcaneus fractures (Sanders type IV) in 6 patients treated with primary subtalar arthrodesis.

▶ Arthrodesis performed through a limited lateral approach and stabilized with 2 or 3 cannulated screws without preliminary calcaneal fracture reduction or fixation.

▶ Average time from injury to surgery: 20 days (15 to 32 days).

▶ Average age: 40 years (18 to 61, 4 males, 4 females).

▶ Follow-up at 2 time points

▷ Short-term average: 12 months (10 to 14 months)

▷ Mid-term average: 52 months (30 to 50 months)

▶ Outcome measurements

▷ AOFAS—maximum score of 94 points due to the lack of inversion and eversion secondary to arthrodesis

▷ Radiographic evaluation

▷ Clinical evaluation

Results

▶ Average AOFAS

▷ 70 points (54 to 84 points) at short-term follow-up

▷ 85 points (78 to 91 points) at medium-term follow-up

▶ Pain

▷ Early follow-up

≫ 3 patients (3 ft) reported mild pain

≫ 2 patients (2 ft) reported no pain

≫ 1 patient (2 ft) reported moderate pain

▷ Mid-term follow-up

>> 2 patients complained of hindfoot pain

>> 4 patients were asymptomatic

▸ All patients were in neutral or valgus alignment on clinical exam.

▸ All patients showed x-ray evidence of subtalar fusion at the short-term follow-up.

Conclusions

▸ The authors concluded that primary subtalar arthrodesis for markedly comminuted Sanders type IV calcaneus fractures yielded good mid-term results.

▸ They also stated that preliminary ORIF of the calcaneus, as recommended by some authors to restore calcaneal height, was not required to obtain good results.

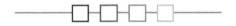

FEATURED ARTICLE
Authors: Radnay CS, Clare MP, Sanders RW.
Title: Subtalar fusion after displaced intra-articular calcaneal fractures: does initial operative treatment matter?
Journal Information: *J Bone Joint Surg Am.* 2009;91(3):541–546.

Study Design: Retrospective Review of a Consecutive Series of Patients

▸ 75 subtalar arthrodesis (in 69 patients) performed for painful post-traumatic subtalar arthritis following a prior displaced intra-articular calcaneus fracture.

▸ 36 calcaneal fractures (34 patients) had initially been treated by ORIF.

▸ Underwent in situ subtalar fusion at an average 22.6 months (9 to 106 months) after ORIF

▷ Average age: 43.1 years (22 to 76 years), 27 males, 7 females

▷ Average follow-up: 62.5 months (48 to 141 months)

▷ 39 calcaneal fractures (35 patients) had initially been treated nonoperatively

▷ Underwent a subtalar distraction arthrodesis at an average 16.4 months (6 to 177 months) after injury

▷ Average age: 46.4 years (25 to 74 years), 25 males, 10 females

▷ Average follow-up: 63.5 months (50 to 122 months)

▸ Outcome measurements

▷ AOFAS Ankle-Hindfoot Scale

▷ MFS

Results

▸ 3 nonunions requiring revision in each group.

▸ Patients who had previously undergone calcaneal ORIF had fewer postop wound complications ($P = .08$)

▷ 11% (4/36) in prior ORIF group

▷ 28% (11/39) in prior nonoperative treatment group

▸ Patients who had previously undergone calcaneal ORIF had significantly higher MFS ($P < .0001$)

▷ MFS 90.8 in prior ORIF group

▷ MFS 79.1 in prior nonoperative treatment group

▸ Group that had previously undergone calcaneal ORIF had significantly higher AOFAS Scores ($P < .0001$)

▷ AOFAS 87.1 in prior ORIF group

▷ AOFAS 73.8 in prior nonoperative treatment group

Conclusions

▸ Initial calcaneal ORIF restores calcaneal shape, alignment, and height, facilitating subsequent subtalar fusion with better long-term functional outcomes.

▸ Compared to patients whose calcaneus fracture was treated nonoperatively, subtalar fusion in patients whose calcaneus fracture was treated with ORIF led to better functional outcomes and fewer wound complications.

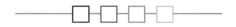

REVIEW ARTICLES

Banerjee R, Chao JC, Taylor R, Siddiqui A. Management of calcaneal tuberosity fractures. *J Am Acad Orthop Surg.* 2012;20(4):253–258.

Buckley RE, Tough S. Displaced intra-articular calcaneal fractures. *J Am Acad Orthop Surg.* 2004;12(3):172–178.

Sanders R. Current concepts review—displaced intra-articular fractures of the calcaneus. *J Bone Joint Surg Am.* 2000;82(2):225–250.

Schepers T. The primary arthrodesis for severely comminuted intra-articular fractures of the calcaneus: a systematic review. *Foot Ankle Surg.* 2012;18(2):84–88.

Lisfranc and Metatarsal Fractures

chapter *2*

FEATURED ARTICLE

Authors: Mologne TS, Lundeen JM, Clapper MF, O'Brien TJ.

Title: Early screw fixation versus casting in the treatment of acute Jones fractures.

Journal Information: *Am J Sports Med.* 2005;33(7):970–975.

Study Design: Prospective, Randomized Study

▸ 37 patients with an acute Jones fracture (fifth metatarsal metaphyseal fractures) in an active duty military population
  ▷ 18 treated nonoperatively
    » Short-leg nonweightbearing cast for 8 weeks, followed by a walking cast or hard-sole shoe until union
  ▷ 19 treated with ORIF
    » Percutaneous 4.5-mm malleolar screw
▸ Average age: 26 years (18 to 58 years), 35 males, 2 females.
▸ Average follow-up: 25 months (15 to 42 months).

Results

▸ Operative treatment
  ▷ 95% (18/19) union in operative treatment group

- ▷ Average time to union in 18 cases that healed: 6.9 weeks (4 to 11 weeks)
- ▷ 1 nonunion requiring bone grafting and repeat fixation to achieve union
- ▷ No refractures
- ▷ No delayed unions
- ▶ Nonoperative treatment
  - ▷ Average time in case: 11 weeks (8 to 17 weeks)
  - ▷ Average time in hard-soled shoe: 3.7 weeks (0 to 19 weeks)
  - ▷ 56% (10/18) union in nonoperative treatment group
  - ▷ Average time to union in 10 cases that successfully healed: 14.5 weeks (8 to 22 weeks)
  - ▷ 8 treatment failures
    - » 5 (28%) nonunions
    - » 1 delayed union that healed at 68 weeks
    - » 2 refractures within first year after original injury

Conclusions

- ▶ High incidence of nonunion, delayed union, and refracture with nonoperative treatment of acute Jones fractures.
- ▶ Long periods of immobilization and nonweightbearing are required to achieve eventual union.
- ▶ Early IM screw fixation is safe and effective, resulting in shorter time to union and faster return to activity.

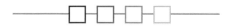

FEATURED ARTICLE
Authors: Ly TV, Coetzee JC.
Title: Treatment of primarily ligamentous Lisfranc joint injuries: primary arthrodesis compared with open reduction and internal fixation. A prospective, randomized study.
Journal Information: *J Bone Joint Surg Am.* 2006;88(3):514–520.

Study Design: Prospective, Randomized Study (Used an Odd or Even Randomization Process, Based on the Order of Presentation)

▸ 41 patients with an isolated acute or subacute primarily ligamentous Lisfranc joint injury

  ▷ 20 patients randomized to ORIF and screw fixation

  ▷ 21 patients randomized to primary arthrodesis of the medial 2 or 3 rays

    » 12 patients had medial 3 rays fused

    » 9 patients had medial 2 rays fused

▸ All patients followed for at least 2 years

  ▷ ORIF group average follow-up: 42 months (25 to 60 months)

  ▷ Primary arthrodesis average follow-up: 43.4 months (25 to 60 months)

▸ Evaluation

  ▷ Clinical examination

  ▷ Radiographs

  ▷ American Orthopaedic Foot and Ankle Society (AOFAS) Midfoot Scale

  ▷ VAS

  ▷ Clinical questionnaire

Results

▸ Anatomic reduction achieved

  ▷ 18/20 patients in ORIF group

  ▷ 20/21 patients in primary arthrodesis group

▸ ORIF group complications

  ▷ 6/20 patients in ORIF group underwent removal of prominent/painful hardware

  ▷ Follow-up x-rays showed loss of correction, increasing deformity, and degenerative joint disease in 15 patients

  ▷ 5 of these patients were subsequently treated with arthrodesis, and 2 more were scheduled for arthrodesis at the time of manuscript preparation

- Primary arthrodesis group complications
  - ▷ 4 patients (19%) had a second surgical procedure, primarily for painful hardware removal
  - ▷ 1 delayed union treated successfully with a bone stimulator
  - ▷ 1 nonunion required bone grafting and revision fusion
  - ▷ 1 patient had a post-traumatic intrinsic compartment syndrome that resulted in claw toes and underwent percutaneous flexor tendon release
- AOFAS Midfoot Scale at 2 years postop (higher score indicates better outcome)
  - ▷ 68.6 points in ORIF group
  - ▷ 88 points in primary arthrodesis group ($P < .005$)
- VAS at final follow-up
  - ▷ 4.1 points in ORIF group
  - ▷ 1.2 points in primary arthrodesis group ($P = .0002$)
- Patients' estimation of their return to physical and sports activity, as a percentage of the preinjury level
  - ▷ 65% in ORIF group at 2-year follow-up
    - » 44% at 6 months, 61% at 1 year, and 65% at 2 years postop
  - ▷ 92% in primary arthrodesis group at 2-year follow-up ($P < .005$)
    - » 62% at 6 months, 86% at 1 year, and 92% at 2 years

Conclusions

- Investigators concluded that treatment of Lisfranc injuries by primary arthrodesis of medial 2 or 3 rays results in better short- and medium-term outcomes compared with traditional ORIF.

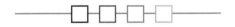

FEATURED ARTICLE

Authors: Henning JA, Jones CB, Sietsema DL, Bohay DR, Anderson JG.

Title: Open reduction internal fixation versus primary arthrodesis for Lisfranc injuries: a prospective randomized study.

Journal Information: *Foot Ankle Int.* 2009;30(10):913–922.

Study Design: Prospective Randomized Study (Randomization by Numbered Envelopes)

- ▶ 40 patients with an acute Lisfranc injury of less than 3 months' duration, no major intra-articular fractures, prior foot pathology, or associated medical comorbidities
  - ▷ 3 dropped out
  - ▷ 5 were lost to follow-up before the 3-month postop visit
- ▶ 32 patients in final group
  - ▷ 14 treated by ORIF
  - ▷ 18 treated by primary fusion
- ▶ Patients evaluated at 3, 6, 12, and 24 months with variable degree of follow-up at each time point
- ▶ Evaluation at 3, 6, 12, and 24 months postop
  - ▷ Clinical examination
  - ▷ Radiographs
  - ▷ SF-36
  - ▷ Short Musculoskeletal Functional Assessment (SMFA)
  - ▷ Overall patient satisfaction phone survey performed

Results

- ▶ ORIF group
  - ▷ 100% anatomic reduction
  - ▷ 11 patients (79%) underwent hardware removal based on standard protocol
  - ▷ 3 patients refused planned hardware removal
  - ▷ 1 patient underwent subsequent arthrodesis
  - ▷ 1 asymptomatic broken screw was noted at 3 months
  - ▷ No infection, loss of fixation, neural injury, or malalignment
  - ▷ At final follow-up, 13 patients (93%) were employed
- ▶ Arthrodesis group
  - ▷ 17 patients (94%) had a solid fusion and anatomic reduction
  - ▷ 3 patients (17%) required additional surgeries for removal of symptomatic hardware
  - ▷ One delayed union with a broken screw healed at 6 months
  - ▷ At final follow-up, 16 patients (89%) were employed
- ▶ Significantly more follow-up surgeries in the ORIF group (79% versus 14%) ($P < .05$)

▸ No statistically significant differences in physical functioning between the 2 groups with regard to SF-36 or SMFA Scores at any follow-up time interval.

▸ No difference in satisfaction rates at an average: 53 months postop.

Conclusions

▸ Primary arthrodesis had significantly fewer secondary surgeries if hardware removal is routinely performed following ORIF.

▸ When performed properly, patients are satisfied with either technique.

▸ No difference in SF-36 or SMFA Scores.

▸ Because of the significant difference in secondary surgeries, and no difference in function, the authors decided to discontinue the study (initially, they planned to enroll 60 patients).

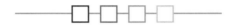

REVIEW ARTICLES

Desmond EA, Chou LB. Current concepts review: Lisfranc injuries. *Foot Ankle Int.* 2006;27(8):653–660.

Rosenberg GA, Sferra JJ. Treatment strategies for acute fractures and nonunions of the proximal fifth metatarsal. *J Am Acad Orthop Surg.* 2000;8(5):332–338.

Schenck RC Jr, Heckman JD. Fractures and dislocations of the forefoot: operative and nonoperative treatment. *J Am Acad Orthop Surg.* 1995;3(2):70–78.

Watson TS, Shurnas PS, Denker J. Treatment of Lisfranc joint injury: current concepts. *J Am Acad Orthop Surg.* 2010;18:(12)718–728.

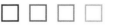

Talus Fractures (Neck, Body, Lateral Process)

chapter 3

CLASSIC ARTICLE
Author: Hawkins LG.
Title: Fractures of the neck of the talus.
Journal Information: *J Bone Joint Surg Am.* 1970;52(5):991–1002.

▸ Classic article that defines the Hawkins classification for talar neck fractures.

Study Design: Retrospective Review

▸ Analyzed 57 consecutive talar neck fractures (55 patients) collected from the University of Iowa (1943 to 1967) and the University of Colorado (1960 to 1969).

▸ Mechanism of injury (forced dorsiflexion)

  ▷ 33 motorcycle or motor vehicle accidents

  ▷ 15 falls from height

  ▷ 5 small plane crashes (true aviator's astragular fractures)

  ▷ 2 crush injuries from object dropped on foot

▸ Developed a classification based on x-ray appearance at time of injury.

Hak DJ.
*Rapid Reference Review in Orthopedic Trauma:
Pivotal Papers Revealed (pp 23-33).*
© 2013 SLACK Incorporated.

Hawkins Classification

- Group I: vertical undisplaced fracture of the talar neck.
- Group II: displaced vertical fracture of talar neck with subluxation or dislocation of subtalar joint but normal ankle joint.
- Group III: displaced vertical talar neck fracture with talus dislocated from both subtalar and ankle joints.
- Note that a fourth type was added by Canale in 1978, which is a group III injury plus dislocation/subluxation of the talonavicular joint.

Results

- Group I
  - ▷ 6 cases
  - ▷ All treated nonoperatively
  - ▷ No cases developed total avascular necrosis (AVN)
  - ▷ No nonunions
- Group II
  - ▷ 24 cases, 3 were open fractures
  - ▷ 10 treated by closed reduction, 14 treated by open reduction
  - ▷ 10 cases developed total AVN
  - ▷ No nonunions
- Group III
  - ▷ 27 cases, 12 were open fractures
  - ▷ 2 treated by closed reduction, 20 treated by open reduction, 5 treated by total talectomy
  - ▷ 20/22 developed total AVN
  - ▷ 3 nonunions

Conclusions

- This historical article also provides a description of "Hawkins sign"
  - ▷ Used to assess talus vascularity between the sixth and eighth week after injury
  - ▷ With nonweightbearing, disuse atrophy is evident on x-ray. AP ankle x-ray reveals the presence or absence of subchondral atrophy in the dome of the talus
  - ▷ Subchondral atrophy excludes the diagnosis of AVN (because bone must be vascularized in order to undergo disuse resorption)

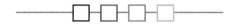

FEATURED ARTICLE

Authors: Canale ST, Kelly FB Jr.

Title: Fractures of the neck of the talus. Long-term evaluation of seventy-one cases.

Journal Information: *J Bone Joint Surg Am.* 1978;60(2):143–156.

▶ This paper first described the type IV talar neck fracture (Hawkins group III plus subluxation/dislocation of talar head from the talonavicular joint).

Study Design: Retrospective Review

▶ 71 talar neck fractures in 70 patients out of a series of 107 fractures treated between 1942 and 1974.
▶ Average patient age at time of fracture: 30 years.
▶ Average follow-up: 12.7 years.
▶ Closed reduction followed by nonweightbearing immobilization was the preferred treatment in mild to moderately displaced fractures.
▶ If an adequate reduction (defined as < 5-mm displacement and < 5 degrees malalignment) was not obtained, open reduction with internal fixation was recommended.
▶ Only 22 patients underwent ORIF.
▶ Used Hawkins scoring system—maximum score 15
  ▷ Pain (none = 6 points, pain on fatigue = 3 points, and so on)
  ▷ Ranges of motion in the ankle and subtalar joints (full = 3 points each, none = 0 points)
  ▷ Limp (none = 3 points)

Results

▶ Overall, 59% had good or excellent results
  ▷ 17 excellent (13 to 15 points)
  ▷ 25 good (10 to 12 points)
  ▷ 11 fair (7 to 9 points)
  ▷ 18 poor (0 to 6 points)

- 52% developed AVN of the talar body
  ▷ 15% (2/13) AVN rate in type I fractures (nondisplaced)
  ▷ 50% AVN (15/30) rate in type II fractures (subluxation or dislocation of the subtalar joint)
  ▷ 84% (16/19) AVN rate in type III fractures (complete dislocation of talar body from subtalar and ankle joint). Note that 4 additional type III cases were treated by Blair fusion or talectomy

Conclusions

- Many patients with avascular necrosis treated conservatively had satisfactory results.
- 25 secondary procedures performed for complications of AVN, malunion, subtalar arthritis, and infection.
- Triple arthrodesis, tibiocalcaneal fusion, and dorsal beak resection of the talar neck all resulted in a high percentage of satisfactory results, but talectomy did not.

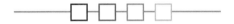

FEATURED ARTICLE

Author: Hawkins LG.

Title: Fracture of the lateral process of the talus: a review of 13 cases.

Journal Information: *J Bone Joint Surg Am.* 1965;47-A:1170–1175.

Study Design: Retrospective Review

- 13 lateral process of talus fractures.
- Not initially recognized on x-rays in 6 cases.
- Described as occurring from a fall from height or motor vehicle accident.

- Mechanism of injury described as forced dorsiflexion of the foot with associated inversion (in contradistinction to subsequent articles, which cite eversion).
- Noted the following 3 types of fractures:
  1. Simple fracture that extends from talofibular articular surface to posterior talocalcaneal articular surface
  2. Comminuted fracture involving both fibular and posterior calcaneal articular surfaces
  3. Chip fracture of anterior and inferior portion of posterior articular process of talus
- Treated by closed reduction and casting in a neutral or everted position.

Results

- 7 patients were pain free and had full motion 8 weeks after injury.
- Pain and disability persisted at 6 months in the other 6 patients requiring operative treatment, either fragment excision or subtalar arthrodesis.

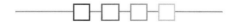

FEATURED ARTICLE

Authors: Vallier HA, Nork SE, Barei DP, Benirschke SK, Sangeorzan BJ.

Title: Talar neck fractures: results and outcomes.

Journal Information: *J Bone Joint Surg Am.* 2004;86-A(8): 1616–1624.

Study Design: Retrospective Review

- 102 talar neck fractures in 100 patients all treated with ORIF.
- Dual (anteromedial and anterolateral) approaches were used in 91 fractures.

- ▶ Fracture classification
  - ▷ Hawkins/Canale
    - » 4 group I
    - » 68 group II
    - » 25 group III
    - » 5 group IV
  - ▷ 24 open fractures (1 type I, 1 type II, 22 type IIIA)
  - ▷ 23 had an associated talar body fracture
  - ▷ 44 had additional ipsilateral foot and ankle injuries
- ▶ 60 fractures (59 patients) were evaluated at average 36-month follow-up (12 to 74 months)
  - ▷ 45 patients had complete functional outcome measurement
  - ▷ 39 had complete radiographs
- ▶ Functional outcome measurement at follow-up (higher scores indicate greater impairment of function)
  - ▷ Foot Functional Index (FFI)
    - » Pain (81 possible points)
    - » Disability (81 possible points)
    - » Activity (45 possible points)
    - » Total score is average of these 3 subscores
    - » Worse outcomes were noted in comminuted fractures ($P < .03$)
  - ▷ Musculoskeletal Function Assessment (MFA)
    - » 10 categories of general health status (100 possible points)
    - » Worse outcomes were noted in comminuted fractures ($P < .03$)

Results

- ▶ Overall AVN rate was 49% (19/39 cases with available radiographs)
  - ▷ 7 showed revascularization of the talar dome without collapse
  - ▷ 31% (12/39) showed collapse of talar dome
  - ▷ AVN occurred within the first 10 months after the injury in all cases
  - ▷ AVN rate was 39% in group II fractures
  - ▷ AVN rate was 64% in group III fractures
  - ▷ AVN rate was 20% in group IV fractures
  - ▷ AVN occurred in 58% (18/31) of patients with talar neck comminution ($P < .03$)

▸ AVN was associated with talar neck comminution and open fractures, confirming that higher-energy injuries are associated with more complications and a worse prognosis.

▸ While attempt was made to fix fractures urgently when patient condition permitted, they found no correlation between the timing of fixation and the development of AVN

  ▷ Average time from injury to ORIF in patients developing AVN was 3.4 days

  ▷ Average time from injury to ORIF in patients without AVN was 5.0 days

▸ Other complication rates

  ▷ 3.3% superficial infection

  ▷ 3.3% wound dehiscence

  ▷ 5.0% deep infection

  ▷ 1.7% delayed union

  ▷ 3.3% nonunion

  ▷ 18% ankle arthritis

  ▷ 15% subtalar arthritis

Conclusions

▸ Fractures of the talar neck are associated with high rates of morbidity and complications.

▸ The authors found no correlation between the timing of fixation and the development of osteonecrosis.

▸ Osteonecrosis was associated with talar neck comminution and open fractures, confirming that higher-energy injuries are associated with more complications and a worse prognosis.

▸ The authors recommended urgent reduction of dislocations and treatment of open injuries and delaying definitive rigid internal fixation until after soft-tissue swelling has subsided in order to minimize soft-tissue complications.

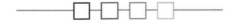

FEATURED ARTICLE
Authors: Vallier HA, Nork SE, Benirschke SK, Sangeorzan BJ.
Title: Surgical treatment of talar body fractures.
Journal Information: *J Bone Joint Surg Am.* 2003;85(9): 1716–1724.

Study Design: Retrospective Review

- 56 patients with 57 talar body fractures treated by ORIF
  - ▷ 23 patients had an associated talar neck fracture
  - ▷ 11 open fractures
- 38 patients were available for follow-up at average 33 months.
- Functional outcome measurement at follow-up (higher scores indicate greater impairment of function)
  - ▷ FFI
  - ▷ MFA
  - ▷ See Valier et al (*J Bone Joint Surg Am.* 2004;86-A[8]:1616–1624) for details of these assessments

Results

- 26 patients had available follow-up radiographs
  - ▷ 88% (23/26) had evidence of AVN and/or post-traumatic arthritis
  - ▷ 10 of 26 patients had AVN of talar body
  - ▷ 5 of 26 had talar dome collapse
- Fractures of both the talar body and neck led to development of advanced arthritis more frequently than did fractures of the talar body only (*P* = .04).
- Worse functional outcomes were noted in association with comminuted and open fractures.
- AVN and post-traumatic arthritis adversely affected outcome scores.

Conclusions

- Talar body ORIF may restore congruity of the adjacent joints; however, early complications are common, and most patients develop radiographic evidence of osteonecrosis and/or post-traumatic arthritis.
- Associated talar neck fractures and open fractures more commonly result in osteonecrosis or advanced arthritis.

▶ Authors emphasized the importance in counseling patients regarding this injury's poor prognosis and potential complications.

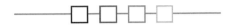

FEATURED ARTICLE
Authors: Valderrabano V, Perren T, Ryf C, Rillmann P, Hintermann B.
Title: Snowboarder's talus fracture: treatment outcome of 20 cases after 3.5 years.
Journal Information: *Am J Sports Med.* 2005;33(6):871–880.

Study Design: Prospective Cohort Study

▶ 20 patients who sustained a lateral process of the talus fracture while snowboarding.

▶ Mechanism of injury: axial-loaded dorsiflexed foot becomes externally rotated and/or everted (in contradistinction to Hawkins earlier presumed mechanism).

▶ The reported injury mechanism included axial impact (100%), dorsiflexion (95%), external rotation (80%), and eversion (45%).

▶ The patients were treated either operatively or nonoperatively based on a fracture-type treatment algorithm.

▶ Fracture classification

▷ 3 type I: chip fractures—all treated nonoperatively

▷ 16 type II: large fragment—14 treated operatively, 2 treated nonoperatively

▷ 1 type III: comminuted—treated nonoperatively

▶ Average follow-up: 42 months (25 to 53 months)

Results

▶ Average American Orthopaedic Foot and Ankle Society (AOFAS) Ankle-Hindfoot Scale was 93 points

▷ Surgically treated group (*n* = 14) scored higher (97 points)

▷ Nonoperative group (*n* = 6; 85 points) (*P* < .05)

- Subtalar joint degenerative osteoarthritis was found in 3 patients (15%)—1 operative and 2 nonoperative patients.
- 16 (80%) patients regained their preinjury level of sporting activity.
- 4 nonoperative cases were unable to return to the same level of sporting activity.

Conclusions

- In type II fractures, primary surgical treatment led to better outcomes and allowed patient to regain his or her preinjury level of sports activity.

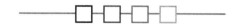

FEATURED ARTICLE
Authors: von Knoch F, Reckord U, von Knoch M, Sommer C.
Title: Fracture of the lateral process of the talus in snowboarders.
Journal Information: *J Bone Joint Surg Br.* 2007;89(6):772–777.

Study Design: Retrospective Review

- 23 consecutive lateral process of the talus fractures in snowboarders.
- Average follow-up: 3.5 years (12 to 76 months).
- 16 treated operatively.
- 7 were minimally displaced and were treated nonoperatively.

Results

- Significant concomitant hindfoot injuries were found in 88% of operative cases.
- Average AOFAS Ankle-Hindfoot Scale: 94 (82 to 100).
- The 7 nonoperative cases with a minimally displaced fracture scored higher (98 points) than the 16 operative cases with displaced or unstable fractures (93 points).

- 65% of patients (10 operative, 5 nonoperative) regained their preinjury level of sporting activity.
- 20 patients were available for x-ray review
  ▷ 45% (9/20) showed subtalar osteoarthritis

Conclusions

- The authors concluded that the outcome after fracture of the lateral process of the talus in snowboarders is favorable as long as an early diagnosis is made and it is adequately treated.
- Treatment recommendation is related to the degree of displacement and associated injuries.

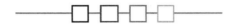

REVIEW ARTICLES

Archdeacon M, Wilber R. Fractures of the talar neck. *Orthop Clin North Am.* 2002;33(1):247–262.

Berkowitz MJ, Kim DH. Process and tubercle fractures of the hindfoot. *J Am Acad Orthop Surg.* 2005;13(8):492–502.

Fortin PT, Balazsy JE. Talus fractures: evaluation and treatment. *J Am Acad Orthop Surg.* 2001;9(2):114–127.

Rammelt S, Zwipp H. Talar neck and body fractures. *Injury.* 2009;40(2):120–135.

Thordarson DB. Talar body fractures. *Orthop Clin North Am.* 2001;32(1):65–77.

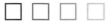

Tibial Pilon Fractures

chapter **4**

CLASSIC ARTICLE
Authors: Rüedi TP, Allgöwer M.
Title: Fractures of the lower end of the tibia into the ankle joint.
Journal Information: *Injury.* 1969;1:92–99.

Study Design: Retrospective Review

▸ 84 consecutive tibial pilon fractures treated by ORIF.

▸ Followed 4 principles of Swiss study group

    1. Reconstruction of correct fibular length

    2. Reconstruction of tibial articular surface

    3. Cancellous autograft of metaphyseal defect

    4. Medial tibial plate fixation

▸ Average age: 39 years (19 to 66 years).

▸ Mechanism of injury

    ▷ 60 skiing injuries

    ▷ 19 falls from a height of 3 to 12 ft or a slip on ice

    ▷ 5 motor vehicle accidents

▸ 5 open injuries.

Hak DJ.
Rapid Reference Review in Orthopedic Trauma:
Pivotal Papers Revealed (pp 35-51).
© 2013 SLACK Incorporated.

- Timing of surgery
  - ▷ 63 operated on the day of injury
  - ▷ 14 delayed 7 days due to severe swelling or "doubtful skin conditions"
  - ▷ 6 treated initially elsewhere with a cast
  - ▷ 1 treated initially elsewhere with an unsuccessful operation
- 3 patients were lost to follow-up, and 1 patient died.
- Average follow-up: 50 months.

Results

- 10 wound healing complications
  - ▷ 4 superficial skin infections
  - ▷ 2 small necrotic skin lesions that healed spontaneously
  - ▷ 1 extensive skin necrosis with associated infection and ankle arthritis
  - ▷ 3 cases of osteomyelitis
- 8 additional operations
  - ▷ 4 ankle arthrodesis for ankle arthritis
  - ▷ 3 osteotomies for varus or valgus deformities
  - ▷ 1 delayed union
- Outcomes
  - ▷ 31 excellent (39%)
  - ▷ 28 good (35%)
  - ▷ 9 moderate (11%)
  - ▷ 12 poor (15%)
  - ▷ 90% able to return to their same occupation
  - ▷ 70% able to return to sports
  - ▷ 57.5% reported pain in bad weather
  - ▷ 48% reported occasional swelling
  - ▷ 48% reported getting tired easily

Conclusions

- The authors concluded that the high percentage of good functional results supported achieving optimal anatomic reconstruction.

Commentary

▸ It is important to note that most patients in this series sustained lower-energy injuries, with only 5 high-energy injuries from motor vehicle accidents. When surgeons in the United States attempted similar treatment for higher-energy injuries, they were unable to produce the same level of good results.

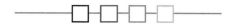

FEATURED ARTICLE

Authors: Sirkin M, Sanders R, DiPasquale T, Herscovici D Jr.

Title: A staged protocol for soft tissue management in the treatment of complex pilon fractures.

Journal Information: *J Orthop Trauma.* 1999;13(2):78–84.

Study Design: Retrospective Review

▸ 56 tibial pilon fractures treated with a 2-stage protocol.

▸ Protocol consisted of immediate (within 24 hours) ORIF of fibula and application of ankle spanning external fixator.

▸ ORIF of tibial pilon was performed when soft-tissue edema resolved, generally at 7 to 14 days after injury.

Results

▸ Follow-up available on 29/30 closed fractures
  ▷ Average time from external fixator to ORIF: 12.7 days (4 to 30 days)
  ▷ 5 cases (17%) developed partial-thickness wound necrosis. All were treated successfully with local wound care
  ▷ 1 late complication of chronic osteomyelitis that resolved with hardware removal
▸ Follow-up available on 17/19 open fractures
  ▷ Average time from external fixator to ORIF: 14 days (4 to 31 days)

▷ 2 cases developed partial-thickness wound necrosis. Both were treated successfully with local wound care

▷ 2 complications (10.5%)

▷ One case (type I open) developed wound dehiscence with deep infection

▷ One case (type IIIA open) with open ipsilateral calcaneus fracture developed severe osteomyelitis in multiple areas and underwent a below knee amputation 5 months after injury

▸ These results compared favorably with the reported historically high rates of infection (11% to 55%) and wound complications (11% to 36%) seen following tibial pilon ORIF.

Conclusions

▸ The authors concluded that the high rate of complications associated with tibial pilon ORIF was due to early operative treatment through swollen compromised soft tissues.

Commentary

▸ This staged protocol presented in this paper, and commonly used today, significantly decreased the complication rates associated with tibial pilon ORIF.

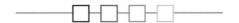

ARTICLE DETAILING COMPLICATIONS OF EARLY TIBIAL PILON ORIF

Authors: Wyrsch B, McFerran MA, McAndrew M, et al.

Title: Operative treatment of fractures of the tibial plafond. A randomized, prospective study.

Journal Information: *J Bone Joint Surg Am.* 1996;78(11):1646–1657.

Study Design: Prospective, Surgeon-Randomized Study of Tibial Pilon Fractures

▶ One group of 2 surgeons performed ORIF of tibial pilon and fibula through 2 incisions (18 patients) or ORIF of tibial pilon alone if fibula intact (one patient).

▶ Second group of 4 surgeons performed external fixation with or without limited internal fixation consisting of fibula plating or tibial interfragmentary screw fixation (20 patients).

▶ 10 (26%) open fractures.

▶ 17 (44%) were Rüedi-Allgöwer-type III fractures.

▶ ORIF group

   ▷ 3 open fractures

   » All treated with emergent irrigation and débridement and ORIF within 5 hours of injury

   ▷ 16 closed fractures

   » ORIF performed within 48 hours unless blisters or severe swelling

   » Average time from injury to operative fixation: 5 days (3 hours to 17 days)

▶ External fixation group

   ▷ 7 open fractures

   ▷ 13 closed fractures

▶ Average follow-up: 39 months (25 to 51 months)

Results

▶ The complications after ORIF tended to be more severe, and amputation was performed in 3 of these cases

   ▷ ORIF group

   » 7 patients had 15 major complications requiring 28 additional operations

   » 6 wound breakdowns requiring free flap coverage

   » 6 deep infections or osteomyelitis

   » 3 amputations

   ▷ External fixation group

   » 4 patients had 4 major complications requiring 5 additional operations

   » 1 partial nerve injury caused by external fixation pin resulting in mild reflex sympathetic dystrophy

» 1 deep infection and failed skin graft requiring free flap

» 1 loss of reduction requiring treatment with thin wire fixator

» 1 pin tract infection subsequently resulting in ankle joint infection requiring 2 débridements and developing spontaneous tibiotalar fusion

▶ Clinical Score (higher score indicated better outcome)

  ▷ Patient questionnaire that evaluated pain and functional outcome

  ▷ Surgeon evaluation of gait and ROM

▶ Clinical Score at the most recent follow-up showed no significant difference between the 2 groups

  ▷ 61 points in ORIF group

  ▷ 72 points in external fixation group

▶ Clinical Scores were worse for type II and type III fractures regardless of the type of treatment.

Conclusions

▶ The investigators concluded that external fixation is a satisfactory method for tibial pilon fractures and is associated with fewer complications than ORIF.

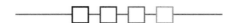

ARTICLE DETAILING COMPLICATIONS OF EARLY TIBIAL PILON ORIF

Authors: McFerran MA, Smith SW, Boulas HJ, Schwartz HS.

Title: Complications encountered in the treatment of pilon fractures.

Journal Information: *J Orthop Trauma*. 1992;6(2):195–200.

This is one of the top 20 cited papers published in the *Journal of Orthopaedic Trauma*, 1987 to 2007.

Study Design: Retrospective Review

▸ 52 tibial pilon fractures in 51 patients treated between 1985 and 1990.

▸ Average age: 40 years (16 to 76 years), 31 males, 21 females.

▸ Average follow-up: 67 weeks (1 to 200 weeks).

▸ Fracture classification

▷ 27% (14/52) Rüedi-Allgöwer type I

▷ 33% (17/52) Rüedi-Allgöwer type II

▷ 40% (21/52) Rüedi-Allgöwer type III

▷ 79% (41/52) closed fractures

▷ 21% (11/52) open fractures

▸ 89% (46/52) underwent ORIF

▷ 2 treated closed

▷ 2 external fixation

▷ 1 fibular ORIF and tibial external fixation

▷ 1 pins and plaster

▸ Average delay from injury to definitive management: 4.7 days (3 hours to 17 days).

▸ Major local complications were defined as those requiring unplanned surgery due to the following:

▷ Infection

▷ Wound breakdown with subsequent flap coverage

▷ Failure of fixation

▷ Failure of fracture healing

Results

▸ 54% overall local complication rate.

▸ 40% (21/52) had major local complications

▷ These major complications required 77 additional surgeries

▷ Major complications occurred in the following:

》 6/14 type I fractures

》 6/17 type II fractures

》 9/21 type III fractures

▸ 10/21 major complications occurred within 3 weeks of ORIF.

▸ Only 2/21 major complications occurred beyond 40 weeks after ORIF.

Conclusions

▸ A surprisingly high complication rate was identified in the treatment of tibial pilon fractures.

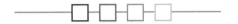

ARTICLE EXAMINING THE SAFETY OF EARLY (NONSTAGED) PILON ORIF

Authors: White TO, Guy P, Cooke CJ, et al.

Title: The results of early primary open reduction and internal fixation for treatment of OTA 43.C-type tibial pilon fractures: a cohort study.

Journal Information: *J Orthop Trauma.* 2010;24(12):757–763.

▸ While most surgeons have advocated a staged approach to fixation of tibial pilon fractures, this group of surgeons reported on a single-stage urgent ORIF of these injuries.

Study Design: Retrospective Review

▸ 115 patients with tibial pilon fractures (AO/OTA 43.C) treated between January 1993 and May 2005

  ▷ Primary ORIF was deemed not possible in 20 cases and was treated with initial external fixation

    ≫ 4 cases were due to local soft-tissue factors

    ≫ 8 cases were due to delayed tertiary transfers

    ≫ 4 cases were due to segmental tibia fractures

    ≫ 4 cases were due to multiple injuries that precluded early complex surgery

  ▷ 95 patients underwent single-stage primary ORIF

  ▷ Primary ORIF was performed within 24 hours of injury in 67 (71%) cases

▷ Primary ORIF was performed within 48 hours of injury in 84 (88%) cases

▷ Median time from injury to ORIF was 18 hours

▸ Average age: 44 years (19 to 68 years).

▸ 1-year minimum follow-up.

▸ Injury mechanism

   ▷ 11 falls from more than 6 m

   ▷ 44 falls from 1 to 3 m

   ▷ 13 falls from < 1 m

   ▷ 21 motor vehicle collisions

   ▷ 5 crush injuries

   ▷ 1 aircraft crash

▸ 21 open fractures

   ▷ 5 type I

   ▷ 7 type II

   ▷ 6 type IIIA

   ▷ 3 type IIIB

▸ Various internal fixation implants, which evolved during the years of the treatment, were used.

▸ Fibula fixed through a lateral approach, and tibia fixed through either an anteromedial or anterolateral surgical approach.

▸ Primary outcome measure: wound dehiscence or deep infection requiring secondary surgery.

▸ Secondary outcome measures

   ▷ Reduction quality

   ▷ Functional outcome as measured by SF-36 and Foot and Ankle Outcome Score

Results

▸ 6 patients (6%) developed wound dehiscence or deep infection requiring surgical débridement

   ▷ 4 were open fractures type IIIA

   ▷ 2 were closed fractures, and both patients had insulin dependent diabetes mellitus

   ▷ 19% (4/21) infection rate in open fractures

   ▷ 2.7% (2/74) infection rate in closed fractures

▸ Anatomic reduction in 90% of cases

Conclusions

▶ The investigators concluded that when surgery is performed expeditiously by experienced trauma surgeons, most tibial pilon fractures can be treated by primary ORIF with outcomes that compare favorably with published reports of other treatment protocols.

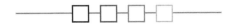

FEATURED ARTICLE

Authors: Wang C, Li Y, Huang L, Wang M.

Title: Comparison of two-staged ORIF and limited internal fixation with external fixator for closed tibial plafond fractures.

Journal Information: *Arch Orthop Trauma Surg.* 2010;130(10): 1289–1297.

Study Design: Prospective Randomized (Based on Odd or Even Numbers) Study

▶ 56 patients with closed type B3 or C pilon fractures
  ▷ 2-staged ORIF (27 cases)
  ▷ Limited internal fixation with external fixation (29 cases)
▶ Outcome measures
  ▷ Bone union
  ▷ Nonunion
  ▷ Malunion
  ▷ Pin-tract infection
  ▷ Wound infection
  ▷ Osteomyelitis
  ▷ Ankle joint function using Mazur Ankle Score (maximum score 100 points, > 87 considered a good-to-excellent result)

Results

▶ No difference in average time to union
  ▷ Average: 25 weeks (12 to 60 weeks) in 2-staged ORIF group
  ▷ Average: 26 weeks (8 to 56 weeks) in limited internal fixation with external fixation group
▶ Significantly fewer superficial soft-tissue infections (either wound or pin-tract) in 2-staged group ($P < .05$).
▶ Higher rates of malunion, delayed union, and arthritis symptoms in the limited internal fixation with external fixation group but differences not significant.
▶ Logistic regression analysis indicated that smoking and fracture pattern were the 2 factors significantly influencing the final outcomes.
▶ No significant difference in Mazur Ankle Scores between the 2 treatment groups
  ▷ 63% (17/27) good-to-excellent in 2-staged ORIF group
  ▷ 55% (16/29) good-to-excellent in limited internal fixation with external fixation group

Conclusions

▶ Both 2-staged ORIF and limited internal fixation with external fixation offer similar results.
▶ Limited internal fixation with external fixation is associated with a higher rate of superficial infections, primarily pin-tract infections, but this does not affect the final outcome.

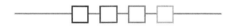

FEATURED ARTICLE
Authors: Pollak AN, McCarthy ML, Bess RS, Agel J, Swiontkowski MF.
Title: Outcomes after treatment of high-energy tibial plafond fractures.
Journal Information: *J Bone Joint Surg.* 2003;85-A(100):1893–1900.

Study Design: Retrospective Cohort Analysis of High-Energy Tibial Pilon Fractures Treated at 2 Centers Between 1994 and 1995

▸ 78% (80/103) of eligible patients completed a follow-up health status evaluation at an average 3.2 years (2 to 5 years)

▷ 70 of these patients also completed a functional status assessment

▸ Patient demographics

▷ Average age at time of follow-up: 44 years (19 to 72 years)

▷ 78% males, 22% females

▷ 64% were at least high school graduates

▷ 79% were insured

▸ Injury characteristics

▷ 61% closed injuries

▷ 74% AO/OTA type C pilon fracture

▷ 8% bilateral pilon fractures

▷ 11% major contralateral lower extremity injury

▸ Included patients treated by ORIF and those treated by external fixation with or without limited internal fixation.

▸ 5 late amputations (4 below knee amputations, 1 above knee amputation)

▷ All had sustained AO/OTA type C fractures

▷ All had been treated by external fixation with limited internal fixation

▷ 4 were initially open injuries

▷ 4 had severe wound infections that required operative treatment before the later amputation

▸ Outcome measurements

▷ SF-36, a general health status assessment

▷ Ambulation Scale of Sickness Impact Profile, to assess lower extremity function

▷ American Medical Association ROM impairment rating

▷ Pain assessed on a 100-point VAS

▷ Stair-climbing performance measured by ability to reciprocally ascend and descend a flight of stairs

Results

- SF-36 Scores were significantly poorer than age- and gender-matched norms.
- 35% reported substantial ankle stiffness.
- 29% reported persistent swelling.
- 33% reported ongoing pain.
- Of 65 patients employed at time of injury, 28 were not employed at follow-up
  - ▷ 68% of those unemployed reported that the pilon fracture prevented them from working
- Multivariable analysis indicated the following factors were related to poorer results:
  - ▷ Presence of 2 or more comorbidities
  - ▷ Being married
  - ▷ Having an annual income less than $25,000
  - ▷ Not having attained a high school diploma
  - ▷ Having been treated with external fixation with or without limited internal fixation

Conclusions

- Investigators concluded that a patient sustaining tibial pilon fractures suffer persistent and devastating consequences to his or her general health and well-being.

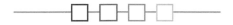

FEATURED ARTICLE

Authors: Marsh JL, Muehling V, Dirschl D, Hurwitz S, Brown TD, Nepola J.

Title: Tibial plafond fractures treated by articulated external fixation: a randomized trial of postoperative motion versus nonmotion.

Journal Information: *J Orthop Trauma.* 2006;20(8):536–541.

Study Design: Prospective, Multicenter, Randomized Trial

- Tibial pilon fractures treated with a hinged external fixator (EBI Medical Systems [Biomet, Warsaw, IN]) and limited internal fixation of the articular surface at 3 level I trauma centers.
- Patients randomized to the following:
  - ▷ Postop ankle motion with a mobile hinge
  - ▷ No motion with a locked hinge
- 55 patients enrolled and randomized into the 2 groups.
- 41 patients completed 1-year follow-up (19 no motion, 22 motion)
  - ▷ Average follow-up of this group: 2.3 years (1 to 5 years)
- 31 patients completed 2-year follow-up (15 no motion, 16 motion).
- Outcome measurements
  - ▷ SF-36
  - ▷ Joint-specific ankle questionnaire
  - ▷ Ankle Osteoarthritis Score (AOS)
  - ▷ ROM

Results

- No significant differences between the 2 groups at either follow-up interval in the ankle ROM, AOS Pain and Disability Scale, or the SF-36 Physical Component Summary (PCS) and Mental Component Summary (MCS) Scales.
- Both groups had lower SF-36 Scores compared to the US normal population.
- Both groups had substantial residual ankle pain and disability based on the AOS.
- Similar rates of adverse events in the 2 groups
  - ▷ 6 patients with adverse events in the no-motion group
  - ▷ 4 patients with adverse events in the motion group
- Patients in the motion group had a longer time in fixator ($P = .008$)
  - ▷ 11.7 weeks average time in fixator in no-motion group
  - ▷ 15.5 weeks average time in fixator in motion group

Conclusions

- The use of long periods of cross joint external fixation that immobilizes the ankle results in similar patient outcomes compared to treatment that incorporates early ankle motion using an articulated hinge.

▶ The authors cautioned, however, that the results should be interpreted with caution because the patient numbers were too small to detect potentially meaningful differences in outcomes and the follow-up was too short to assess for differences in the development of arthrosis.

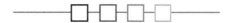

FEATURED ARTICLE

Authors: Tornetta P III, Weiner L, Bergman M, et al.

Title: Pilon fractures: treatment with combined internal and external fixation.

Journal Information: *J Orthop Trauma.* 1993;7(6):489–496.

This is one of the top 20 cited papers published in the *Journal of Orthopaedic Trauma*, 1987 to 2007.

Study Design: Prospective Cohort Study

▶ 26 patients with distal tibial fractures treated with limited internal fixation and the application of a hybrid external fixator (tensioned wires distally and 5.0-mm half pins proximally attached to a semicircular frame without crossing the ankle joint).

▶ Average age: 32 years (15 to 55 years).

▶ Patients followed for 8 to 36 months.

▶ Fracture classification

　▷ 17 intra-articular tibial pilon fractures

　　» 1 Rüedi-Allgöwer type 1

　　» 3 Rüedi-Allgöwer type 2

　　» 13 Rüedi-Allgöwer type 3

　▷ 9 extra-articular distal tibia fractures

　▷ 6 open fractures

▶ 11/17 intra-articular fractures had bone grafting.

▸ Clinical outcome assessment

▷ Excellent: No pain, dorsiflexion > 5 degrees, plantarflexion > 40 degrees, angulation < 3 degrees

▷ Good: Intermittent pain relieved by nonsteroidal anti-inflammatory drugs, dorsiflexion 0 to 5 degrees, plantar flexion 30 to 40 degrees, angulation 3 to 5 degrees valgus or < 3 degrees varus

▷ Fair: Pain with activities of daily living relieved by narcotics, dorsiflexion –5 to 0 degrees, plantarflexion 25 to 30 degrees, angulation 5 to 8 degrees valgus or 3 to 5 degrees varus

▷ Poor: Intractable pain, dorsiflexion < –5 degrees, plantarflexion < 25 degrees, angulation > 8 degrees valgus or > 5 degrees varus

Results

▸ Average time to union: 4.2 months (3 to 7 months).

▸ 81% overall good and excellent results

▷ 13 excellent

▷ 8 good

▷ 3 fair

▷ 2 poor

▸ Results by specific fracture type

▷ Extra-articular

» 7 excellent

» 2 good

▷ Rüedi-Allgöwer type I

» 1 excellent

▷ Rüedi-Allgöwer type II

» 1 excellent

» 1 good

» 1 fair

▷ Rüedi-Allgöwer type III

» 4 excellent

» 5 good

» 2 fair

» 2 poor

▶ Complications
  ▷ 1 superficial infection
  ▷ 1 deep infection
  ▷ 1 10-degree varus malunion
  ▷ 3 pin tract infections

Conclusions

▶ This method yielded results comparable to previous studies while reducing the amount of soft-tissue dissection necessary for the placement of large plates.
▶ Soft-tissue complications were infrequent.
▶ The goals of early motion and fracture stability were not sacrificed.

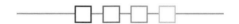

REVIEW ARTICLES

Crist BD, Khazzam M, Murtha YM, Della Rocca GJ. Pilon fractures: advances in surgical management. *J Am Acad Orthop Surg.* 2011;19(10):612–622.

Papadokostakis G, Kontakis G, Giannoudis P, Hadjipavlou A. External fixation devices in the treatment of fractures of the tibial plafond: a systematic review of the literature. *J Bone Joint Surg Br.* 2008;90(1):1–6.

Tarkin IS, Clare MP, Marcantonio A, Pape HC. An update on the management of high-energy pilon fractures. *Injury.* 2008;39(2):142–154.

Thordarson DB. Complications after treatment of tibial pilon fractures: prevention and management strategies. *J Am Acad Orthop Surg.* 2000;8(4):253–265.

Ankle Fractures

chapter **5**

Study Design: Cadaveric Study

▸ Examined effect of lateral talar shift on ankle joint contact area in 23 lower extremity amputation specimens.

▸ Removed fibula and soft tissues.

▸ Measured talus contact in the following positions:

  ▷ Normal articular

  ▷ 1 mm of lateral displacement

  ▷ 2 mm of lateral displacement

  ▷ 4 mm of lateral displacement

  ▷ 6 mm of lateral displacement

▸ Used powdered black carbon to measure contact area during an axially directed load of 70 kg.

Results

▸ 42% average decrease in contact area with 1 mm of lateral talar shift.

Hak DJ.
Rapid Reference Review in Orthopedic Trauma:
Pivotal Papers Revealed (pp 53-70).
© 2013 SLACK Incorporated.

- Additional 14% average decrease in contact area with an additional lateral shift to 2 mm.
- Additional 9% average decrease in contact area with an additional lateral shift to 4 mm.
- Additional 3% average decrease in contact area with an additional lateral shift to 6 mm.
- Tibiotalar contact areas with varying amount of lateral displacement
  - ▷ No lateral talar displacement
    - » 4.40 cm^2 average tibiotalar contact area (range 2.3 to 6.7 cm^2)
  - ▷ 1 mm lateral talar displacement
    - » 2.50 cm^2 average tibiotalar contact area (range 1.0 to 5.0 cm^2)
  - ▷ 2 mm lateral talar displacement
    - » 1.89 cm^2 average tibiotalar contact area (range 1.1 to 3.3 cm^2)
  - ▷ 4 mm lateral talar displacement
    - » 1.53 cm^2 average tibiotalar contact area (range 0.9 to 3.0 cm^2)
  - ▷ 6 mm lateral talar displacement
    - » 1.37 cm^2 average tibiotalar contact area (range 0.7 to 2.5 cm^2)

Conclusions

- Because stress per unit area increases as the total contact area decreases, the decrease in tibiotalar contact area may contribute to poor outcomes following ankle fractures when lateral talar displacement is more than 1 mm.

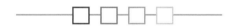

FEATURED ARTICLE
Authors: Boden SD, Labropoulos PA, McCowin P, Lestini WF, Hurwitz SR.
Title: Mechanical considerations for the syndesmosis screw. A cadaver study.
Journal Information: *J Bone Joint Surg Am.* 1989;71(10):1548–1555.

Study Design

▸ This cadaveric study attempted to determine which ankle fractures require syndesmotic fixation.

▸ Pronation external rotation load applied to 25 cadaveric specimens

   ▷ In group I, the deltoid ligament, syndesmosis, and interosseous membrane were serially sectioned in 1.5-cm increments

   ▷ In group II, the deltoid ligament was kept intact, and a medial malleolar osteotomy was performed. After reduction and testing, the deltoid ligament was transected

Results

▸ Group I: deltoid ligament transected and fixation only of fibula fracture

   ▷ Average syndesmotic widening increased gradually from 0.5 to 4.5 mm as the level of fibular fracture rose from 1.5 to 15 cm proximal to the ankle

▸ Group II: deltoid ligament intact and fixation of both medial malleolus and fibula

   ▷ Only minimum syndesmotic widening (1.4 ± 0.3 mm) occurred, even when the fibular fracture was 15 cm proximal to the ankle

   ▷ Then, when the deltoid ligament was sectioned, the average maximum syndesmotic widening was equivalent to that seen in group I

Conclusions

▸ Considering the range of clinically acceptable widening of the syndesmosis, the critical transition zone for the level of a fibular fracture that is fixed with a plate is 3 to 4.5 cm proximal to the ankle.

▸ When the fibular fracture is proximal to this level and rigid medial fixation is not possible, the syndesmosis may have to be stabilized to supplement the fixation with the plate.

▸ However, rigid medial and lateral fixation should acceptably stabilize the syndesmosis without further additional supplementation.

Commentary

▸ While frequently quoted, all of the conclusions of this cadaveric study are not universally accepted. Rigid medial and lateral fixation may not always acceptably stabilize the syndesmosis. Instead, the syndesmosis should be manually checked following any fibula fixation as the severity of the soft-tissue disruption and associated injuries may require syndesmotic fixation even when the fracture is within 3 to 4.5 cm of the ankle joint.

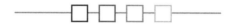

FEATURED ARTICLE

Authors: Pakarinen H, Flinkkilä T, Ohtonen P, et al.

Title: Intraoperative assessment of the stability of the distal tibiofibular joint in supination-external rotation injuries of the ankle: sensitivity, specificity, and reliability of two clinical tests.

Journal Information: *J Bone Joint Surg Am.* 2011;93(22): 2057–2061.

Study Design: Prospective Cohort Study

▸ 140 patients with an unstable unilateral ankle fracture resulting from a supination-external rotation mechanism.

▸ After internal fixation of the malleolar fracture, a hook test and a clinical external rotation stress test were performed independently by the lead surgeon and assisting surgeon, followed by a standardized 7.5-Nm external rotation stress test of each ankle under fluoroscopy.

▸ A positive stress test result was defined as a side-to-side difference of > 2 mm in the tibiotalar or the tibiofibular clear space on mortise radiographs.

▸ The sensitivity and specificity of each test were calculated with use of the standardized 7.5-Nm external rotation stress test as a reference.

Results

▸ 24 (17%) of the 140 patients had a positive standardized 7.5-Nm external rotation stress test after internal fixation of the malleolar fracture.

▸ Hook test had a sensitivity of 0.25 (95% confidence interval [CI]: 0.12 to 0.45) and a specificity of 0.98 (95% CI: 0.94 to 1.0) for the detection of the same instabilities.

▸ Clinical external rotation stress test had a sensitivity of 0.58 (95% CI: 0.39 to 0.76) and a specificity of 0.96 (95% CI: 0.90 to 0.98).

▸ Both tests had excellent interobserver reliability, with 99% agreement for the hook test and 98% for the stress test.

Conclusions

▸ Interobserver agreement for the hook test and the clinical stress test was excellent.

▸ The specificity of both the hook test and the clinical stress test was excellent.

▸ However, the sensitivity was poor for the hook test and only fair for the clinical stress test when a standardized 7.5-Nm external rotation stress test was used as the reference to indicate syndesmotic instability.

Commentary

▸ The variability in performance of tests to examine syndesmotic instability is highlighted in this paper. Examiners commonly use force less than the 7.5-Nm force used in the standardized test. Because stabilization of syndesmotic instability is felt to be essential for optimal long-term outcomes following ankle fractures, the poor sensitivity of these commonly used tests suggests that some patients with syndesmotic instability may not be accurately diagnosed intraoperatively, leading to late instability, pain, and arthritis.

▸ The high specificity of these common tests indicates that these tests prevent unnecessary syndesmotic fixation.

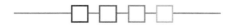

FEATURED ARTICLE

Authors: Wikerøy AK, Høiness PR, Andreassen GS, Hellund JC, Madsen JE.

Title: No difference in functional and radiographic results 8.4 years after quadricortical compared with tricortical syndesmosis fixation in ankle fractures.

Journal Information: *J Orthop Trauma.* 2010;24(1):17–23.

Study Design: This Is a Longer-Term Follow-Up Study of Patients Reported in Their Randomized Study Comparing Tricortical Versus Quadricortical Syndesmotic Fixation (Høiness, Strømsøe. J Orthop Trauma. 2004;18[6]:331–337).

▸ Long-term follow-up is available on 48 of 64 patients studied in their original prospective randomized study

  ▷ 23 quadricortical syndesmotic fixation

  ▷ 25 tricortical syndesmotic fixation

▸ Average follow-up: 8.4 years (7.7 to 8.9 years).

Results

▸ No statistical differences in the 2 groups regarding Olerud and Molander Ankle Score, OTA Score, or degree of osteoarthritis.

▸ Patients with a difference in the syndesmotic width between the operated and the nonoperated ankle of 1.5 mm or more showed a tendency toward poorer functional results ($P = .056$).

▸ Patients with a posterior fracture fragment had a poorer Olerud and Molander Ankle Score (73.1 versus 85, $P = .05$).

▸ 100% of patients with a posterior fracture fragment had osteoarthritis compared with 55% of those without a posterior fragment.

▸ Obese patients (body mass index greater than 30 kg/m^2) also had poorer OTA Score, but neither obesity nor being overweight predicted late arthritis.

Conclusions

▸ Both tricortical and quadricortical syndesmotic fixation showed satisfactory functional results with only minor differences.

▸ Obese patients had significantly poorer functional results.

▸ The presence of a posterior fracture fragment was an important negative prognostic factor regarding functional results.

▸ A difference in syndesmotic width 1.5 mm or greater between the 2 ankles seemed to be associated with an inferior clinical result.

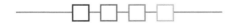

FEATURED ARTICLE

Authors: Høiness P, Strømsøe K.

Title: Tricortical versus quadricortical syndesmosis fixation in ankle fractures: a prospective, randomized study comparing two methods of syndesmosis fixation.

Journal Information: *J Orthop Trauma.* 2004;18(6):331–337.

Study Design: Prospective Randomized Study

▸ Tricortical versus quadricortical syndesmotic fixation.
▸ 64 patients with unstable ankle syndesmosis
  ▷ 30 treated with 1 4.5-mm cortical screw placed through both tibial cortices (quadricortical)
    » Quadricortical screw routinely removed after 2 months
  ▷ 34 treated with 2 3.5-mm cortical screws that engaged only one tibial cortex (tricortical)
    » Tricortical screws were removed only in cases of discomfort

Results

▸ At 3 months, the Olerud and Molander Functional Score (0 to 100) was significantly higher in the tricortical group ($P = .025$)
  ▷ Tricortical group: 77 points
  ▷ Quadricortical group: 66 points
▸ At 1 year, there was no statistical difference in the Olerud and Molander Functional Score ($P = .192$)
  ▷ Tricortical group: 93 points
  ▷ Quadricortical group: 86 points
▸ At 3 months, pain was significantly lower in the tricortical group ($P = .017$).
▸ At 1 year, there was no significant difference in pain between the 2 groups.
▸ No significant difference in dorsiflexion between the groups at any time point.

Conclusions

▶ Syndesmosis fixation with 2 tricortical screws is safe and improves early function.

▶ However, after 1 year, there were no significant differences between tricortical and quadricortical syndesmotic fixation in functional score, pain, and dorsiflexion.

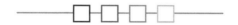

FEATURED ARTICLE

Authors: Makwana NK, Bhowal B, Harper WM, Hui AW.

Title: Conservative versus operative treatment for displaced ankle fractures in patients over 55 years of age. A prospective, randomized study.

Journal Information: *J Bone Joint Surg Br.* 2001;83(4):525–529.

Study Design: Prospective Randomized Study

▶ ORIF with closed reduction compared to cast immobilization of displaced ankle fractures.

▶ All patients > 55 years, average age: 66 years (55 to 81 years)

  ▷ Osteoporosis and older age had been cited as a reason to avoid ORIF

▶ Used specific criteria for satisfactory closed reduction (3 patients were excluded from the study for unsatisfactory closed reduction).

▶ 43 patients randomized

  ▷ 22 ORIF

  ▷ 21 closed treatment

▶ Assessment

  ▷ Clinical evaluation

  ▷ Radiographic evaluation

▷ Olerud and Molander Functional Outcome Score

  » Includes pain, function, swelling, and stiffness

▷ VAS pain

▸ 36 patients evaluated at an average follow-up: 27 months (15 to 42 months).

Results

▸ Closed treatment resulted in significantly less reliable anatomical reduction (P = .03).

▸ Closed treatment resulted in significantly more common loss of reduction (P = .001).

▸ No difference in VAS Pain Score.

▸ ORIF resulted in a significantly higher Olerud and Molander Score (P = .03).

▸ ORIF resulted in a significantly better ankle ROM; (P = .044)

  ▷ ORIF group: ROM within 9 degrees of uninjured side

  ▷ Closed group: ROM within 16 degrees of uninjured side

Conclusions

▸ Authors recommend ORIF of displaced ankle fractures even in older patients.

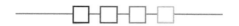

FEATURED ARTICLE

Authors: Lehtonen H, Järvinen TL, Honkonen S, Nyman M, Vihtonen K, Järvinen M.

Title: Use of a cast compared with a functional ankle brace after operative treatment of an ankle fracture. A prospective, randomized study.

Journal Information: *J Bone Joint Surg Am.* 2003;85-A(2): 205–211.

Study Design: Prospective Randomized Study

▸ 100 patients with an unstable and/or displaced Weber type A or B ankle fracture treated operatively.

▸ Randomized to treatment for 6 weeks postop either by:

  ▷ Immobilization in a below-the-knee cast (50 patients)

  ▷ Early mobilization in a functional ankle brace (50 patients)

▸ Outcome measurements

  ▷ Clinical examination

  ▷ Radiographic examination

  ▷ Olerud and Molander Score

  ▷ Kaikkonen Scale

▸ Average age: 41 years, 56 males, 44 females

▸ Follow-up

  ▷ 12 patients were lost to follow-up before the 2-year follow-up exam

  ▷ 42 patients in cast group completed 2-year follow-up

  ▷ 46 patients in functional brace group completed 2-year follow-up

Results

▸ No perioperative complications in either group.

▸ Significantly more postop complications in the functional brace group (P = .0005)

  ▷ 8 (16%) postop complications in cast group

    ≫ 4 superficial wound infections treated with oral antibiotics

    ≫ 2 DVTs

    ≫ 1 chronic skin irritation

    ≫ 1 chronic skin dysesthesia

  ▷ 33 (66%) postop complications in functional brace group

    ≫ 16 superficial wound infections treated with oral antibiotics

    ≫ 4 deep wound infections treated with IV antibiotics

    ≫ 3 wound dehiscences

    ≫ 3 chronic dysesthesias

    ≫ 2 chronic skin irritations

    ≫ 1 local skin necrosis

    ≫ 1 chronic allodynia

    ≫ 1 loss of fixation

    ≫ 1 refracture

    ≫ 1 postspinal headache

▸ No significant differences between the 2 groups in final subjective or objective evaluation.

▸ Average Olerud and Molander Score showed no significant difference at 2 years

  ▷ Cast group 87 ± 8 points

  ▷ Functional brace group 87 ± 9 points

▸ Average Kaikkonen Ankle-Rating Scale showed no significant difference at 2 years

  ▷ Cast group 85 ± 9 points

  ▷ Functional brace group 83 ± 10 points

Conclusions

▸ Postop treatment of ankle fractures with a cast or a functional brace has similar long-term functional outcomes.

▸ While early mobilization with use of a functional ankle brace may have some theoretical beneficial effects, the risk of postop wound complications is considerably increased compared with cast treatment.

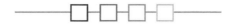

FEATURED ARTICLE

Authors: DeAngelis NA, Eskander MS, French BG.

Title: Does medial tenderness predict deep deltoid ligament incompetence in supination-external rotation type ankle fractures?

Journal Information: *J Orthop Trauma.* 2007;21(4):244–247.

Study Design: Prospective Cohort Study

▸ 55 patients with Weber B ankle fractures and a normal medial clear space on standard plain radiographs.

▸ Average age: 42 years (16 to 78 years), 26 males, 29 females.

▸ Patients were examined for the presence of tenderness to palpation in the region of the deltoid ligament.

▶ Patients then underwent an external rotation stress mortise view radiograph.

Results

▶ 26 patients (47.3%) had medial tenderness
  ▷ 13 patients (23.6%) were tender medially and had a positive external rotation stress test
  ▷ 13 patients (23.6%) were tender medially and had a negative external rotation stress test
▶ 29 patients (52.7%) were not tender medially
  ▷ 19 patients (34.5%) were not tender medially and had a negative external rotation stress test
  ▷ 10 patients (18.2%) were not tender medially and had a positive external rotation stress test
▶ No association between medial tenderness and deep deltoid ligament incompetence (χ^2 = 2.39, P = .12).
▶ Medial tenderness as a measure of deep deltoid ligament incompetence
  ▷ Sensitivity 57%
  ▷ Specificity 59%
  ▷ Positive predictive value 50%
  ▷ Negative predictive value 66%
  ▷ Accuracy 42%

Conclusions

▶ In patients with normal clear space on standard plain radiographs, medial tenderness cannot be used to accurately assess the potential for deep deltoid ligament incompetence.

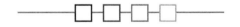

FEATURED ARTICLE

Authors: McConnell T, Creevy W, Tornetta P III.

Title: Stress examination of supination external rotation-type fibular fractures.

Journal Information: *J Bone Joint Surg Am.* 2004;86-A(10): 2171–2178.

Study Design: Prospective Cohort Study

- Patients with Weber B ankle fractures evaluated for tenderness, ecchymosis, and swelling.
- Stress radiographs were performed on patients with isolated fibula fractures and an intact mortise to differentiate supination external rotation-2 (SE2) from supination external rotation-4 (SE4) injury patterns.
- Patients with SE2 patterns were treated nonoperatively and were allowed immediate full weight bearing in an air stirrup brace.

Results

- 97 patients presented with isolated fibular fracture and intact mortise
  - ▷ 61 had a negative stress exam (stable SE2 injury)
  - ▷ 36 had a positive stress exam (SE4 injury)
- Medial tenderness, ecchymosis, and swelling were not predictive of deltoid incompetence
  - ▷ Positive predictive value of severe medial tenderness in predicting instability was only 56%
  - ▷ Negative predictive value of no or mild medial tenderness in predictive stability was 69%

Conclusions

- Soft-tissue indicators are not accurate predictors of instability in Weber B ankle fractures.
- Stress radiographs provide accurate diagnosis of deltoid ligament incompetence.

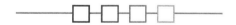

FEATURED ARTICLE
Authors: Donken CC, Verhofstad MH, Edwards MJ, van Laarhoven CJ.
Title: Twenty-one-year follow-up of supination-external rotation type II-IV (OTA type B) ankle fractures: a retrospective cohort study.
Journal Information: *J Orthop Trauma.* 2012;26(8):e108–e114.

Study Design: Retrospective Cohort Study

▸ Long-term follow-up of 148 patients who had sustained a supination external rotation (SER) type II, III, or IV ankle fracture between 1985 and 1990

▷ Represents 54% of all SER II to IV ankle fractures treated during that time

▷ 76 SER-II injuries: 53 treated nonoperatively and 23 treated operatively

▷ 4 SER-III injuries: 2 treated nonoperatively and 2 treated operatively

▷ 68 SER-IV injuries: 61 treated operatively and 7 treated nonoperatively

▸ Median follow-up 21.1 years (17.3 to 23.7 years).

▸ Outcome measurements

▷ Olerud and Molander Score (functional outcome)

▷ ROM

▷ Functional impairment (American Medical Association [AMA] guidelines)

▷ Radiologic evaluation

» Cedell Anatomic Score

» Medial clear space widening

» Presence of osteoarthritis

Results

▸ 92% had a good or excellent Olerud and Molander Score

▷ Overall median Olerud and Molander Score 95 (5 to 100)

▷ SER-II median Olerud and Molander Score 100 (35 to 100)

▷ SER-III median Olerud and Molander Score 100 (85 to 100)

▷ SER-IV median Olerud and Molander Score 95 (5 to 100)

▸ 97% had good or excellent ROM.

▸ 92% had medial clear space widening ≤1 mm.

▸ 76% had good or excellent Cedell Anatomic Score.

▸ 79% had either no signs of arthritis or had osteophytes without evidence of joint space narrowing.

▸ Functional impairment as a percentage of whole-person impairment ranged from 0% to 1%.

▸ Outcomes of operatively and nonoperatively treated SER-II injuries were equivalent on all parameters.

▸ SER-IV injuries had worse outcomes compared to SER-II and SER-III injuries (except for ROM).

Conclusions

▸ Long-term overall results of surgical treatment of SER type II to IV ankle fractures are excellent or good in the majority of patients.

▸ Long-term overall results of nonoperative treatment of SER type II ankle fractures are excellent or good in the majority of patients.

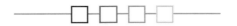

FEATURED ARTICLE

Authors: Donken CC, Verhofstad MH, Edwards MJ, van Laarhoven CJ.

Title: Twenty-two-year follow-up of pronation-external rotation type III-IV (OTA type C) ankle fractures: a retrospective cohort study.

Journal Information: *J Orthop Trauma.* 2012;26(8):e115–e122.

Study Design: Retrospective Cohort Study

▸ Long-term follow-up of 60 patients who had sustained a pronation external rotation (PER) type III or IV ankle fracture between 1985 and 1990

▷ 4 true PER-II injuries: 2 treated nonoperatively and 2 treated operatively

▷ 5 unclear injuries (between PER-III and IV): 2 treated nonoperatively and 3 treated operatively

▷ 51 PER-IV injuries: 46 treated operatively and 5 treated nonoperatively

▸ Treatment protocol

▷ Stable fractures with tibiotalar congruity were treated nonoperatively

▷ Unstable and displaced fractures were treated operatively

- Median follow-up 21.6 years (range 19.3 to 23.7 years)
- Outcome measurements
  ▷ Olerud and Molander Score (functional outcome)
  ▷ ROM
  ▷ Functional impairment (AMA guidelines)
  ▷ Radiologic evaluation
    » Cedell Anatomic Score
    » Medial clear space widening
    » Presence of osteoarthritis

Results

- 90% had a good or excellent Olerud and Molander Score
  ▷ Overall median Olerud and Molander Score 98 (20 to 100)
  ▷ SER-II median Olerud and Molander Score 100 (35 to 100)
  ▷ SER-III median Olerud and Molander Score 100 (85 to 100)
  ▷ SER-IV median Olerud and Molander Score 95 (5 to 100)
- 88% had good or excellent ROM.
- 85% had medial clear space widening of 1 mm or less.
- 78% had either no signs of arthritis or had osteophytes without evidence of joint space narrowing.
- 83% had good or excellent Cedell Anatomic Score.
- Functional impairment as a percentage of whole-person impairment ranged from 0% to 3%.
- Patients treated operatively and nonoperatively had statistically equivalent scores.
- A subgroup analysis showed no difference in patients treated with syndesmotic fixation alone compared to those treated with syndesmotic fixation in combination with fibular plate fixation.
- 18 patients had bone bridging between the fibula and tibia.
- Patients with and without bone bridging had equivalent scores.

Conclusions

- The long-term results of surgical treatment of PER ankle fractures are good or excellent in the majority of patients.

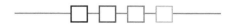

FEATURED ARTICLE

Authors: Sanders DW, Tieszer C, Corbett B; and Canadian Orthopedic Trauma Society.

Title: Operative versus nonoperative treatment of unstable lateral malleolar fractures: a randomized multicenter trial.

Journal Information: *J Orthop Trauma*. 2012;26(3):129–134.

Study Design: Prospective, Randomized, Multicenter Study

▶ 81 patients with isolated fibula fractures (Weber B) without evidence of talar shift on injury radiographs but with evidence of instability on stress radiographs

  ▷ Instability is defined as the following:

   » 1 mm or more increase in medial clear space (medial edge of talar dome to lateral edge of medial malleolus)

   » Absolute medial clear space 5 mm or more

▶ Randomized to operative versus nonoperative treatment

  ▷ 41 patients underwent ORIF treatment using a lag screw (when possible) and fibular stabilization with neutralization or an antiglide plate

  ▷ 40 patients were treated nonoperatively with a plaster or fiberglass cast or brace

  ▷ Both groups had protected weightbearing for 6 weeks

▶ Outcome measurements

  ▷ Olerud and Molander Ankle Score

  ▷ SF-36

  ▷ Radiographic evaluation

Results

▶ No statistically significant differences in functional outcome scores or pace of recovery between the operative and nonoperative groups.

▶ Complications

  ▷ Nonoperative group

   » 8 radiographic misalignment—defined as medial clear space of 5 mm or more

   » 8 delayed union or nonunion

▷ Operative group
  » 5 surgical site infections
  » 5 required hardware removal

Conclusions

▸ Satisfactory functional outcome and pace of recovery were achieved with both operative and nonoperative treatment.

▸ Radiographic results were superior in the operative group with less risk of delayed union and substantially less risk of misalignment.

▸ Based on their results, they recommended that older and less active individuals are safely treated nonoperatively with equivalent functional outcomes.

▸ In younger patients, the observed risk of misalignment supports consideration of operative intervention.

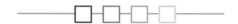

REVIEW ARTICLES

Chaudhary SB, Liporace FA, Gandhi A, Donley BG, Pinzur MS, Lin SS. Complications of ankle fracture in patients with diabetes. *J Am Acad Orthop Surg.* 2008;16(3):159–170.

Michelson JD. Ankle fractures resulting from rotational injuries. *J Am Acad Orthop Surg.* 2003;11(6):403–412.

Wuest TK. Injuries to the distal lower extremity syndesmosis. *J Am Acad Orthop Surg.* 1997;5(3):172–181.

Tibial Shaft Fractures

chapter 6

FEATURED ARTICLE

Authors: Bone LB, Kassman S, Stegemann P, France J.

Title: Prospective study of union rate of open tibial fractures treated with locked, unreamed intramedullary nails.

Journal Information: *J Orthop Trauma.* 1994;8(1):45–49.

This is one of the top 20 cited papers published in the *Journal of Orthopaedic Trauma*, 1987 to 2007.

Study Design: Prospective Nonrandomized Study of 29 Consecutive Patients

▸ Objective was to see whether open tibial fractures would heal following unreamed tibial nailing without bone grafting.

▸ Evaluated with x-rays at monthly intervals.

▸ Average age: 31 years (16 to 80 years).

▸ 27 were open fractures.

▸ 2 additional fractures were "open by surgical intent"—closed fractures with compartment syndrome requiring fasciotomy.

▸ Open fracture grading

  ▷ 16 type I

  ▷ 8 type II

  ▷ 3 type IIIA

Hak DJ.
Rapid Reference Review in Orthopedic Trauma: Pivotal Papers Revealed (pp 71-88).
© 2013 SLACK Incorporated.

- Fracture pattern
  - ▷ 22 comminuted or segmental
  - ▷ 7 noncomminuted
- Interlocking
  - ▷ 15 dynamically interlocked
  - ▷ 14 statically interlocked
- Secondary surgery was considered if there was no evidence of bridging callus between 3 and 6 months postop.

Results

- 15 fractures healed without secondary surgical intervention.
- 14 fractures required from 1 to 3 (average 1.9) additional surgeries to achieve union
  - ▷ 3 dynamization (removal of static interlocking screws)
  - ▷ 2 exchange reamed nailing
  - ▷ 2 iliac crest bone grafting
  - ▷ 7 patients had varying combination of procedures during 13 additional procedures
    - » Dynamization (3 patients)
    - » Exchange reamed nailing (4 patients)
    - » Fibular osteotomy (4 patients)
    - » Bone grafting (8 patients)
- Average time to union: 148 days.
- Rate of secondary surgery was significantly higher in comminuted fractures ($P < .001$)
  - ▷ 7/7 noncomminuted fractures did not require secondary intervention
  - ▷ 13/22 comminuted fractures required secondary intervention

Conclusions

- The authors concluded that unreamed nailing did not improve union rates compared to the historical rate for external fixation.
- They recommended a treatment algorithm for open tibial fracture treated with unreamed IM nailing based on whether the fracture pattern is stable or unstable
  - ▷ Stable fracture patterns
    - » Treated with dynamic interlocking
    - » Patients remain partial weightbearing until axially stable (usually about 6 to 8 weeks)
    - » If delayed union develops, perform bone grafting at 4 to 6 months

▷ Unstable fracture patterns

» Treated with static interlocking

» Dynamize when axially stable (usually about 6 to 8 weeks) and if indicated, also consider early bone grafting

» If delayed union develops, perform bone grafting at 4 to 6 months

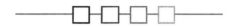

FEATURED ARTICLE
Authors: Sarmiento A, Latta LL.
Title: Fractures of the middle third of the tibia treated with a functional brace.
Journal Information: *Clin Orthop Relat Res.* 2008;466(12): 3108–3115.

Study Design: Retrospective Review

▶ 434 closed middle third diaphyseal tibial fractures treated with a functional brace.

▶ Average follow-up: 4.3 months (1.5 to 14.3 months).

Results

▶ 97% of middle third fractures healed with 8 degrees or less angulation in the mediolateral plane.

▶ Average final shortening: 4.3 mm.

▶ 4 (0.9%) patients developed nonunion.

▶ Found correlations between initial shortening and final shortening, initial displacement and final displacement, and time to brace with initial angulation and final angulation in the mediolateral and AP planes.

Conclusions

▶ Satisfactory results can be obtained in most instances using a functional brace for management of closed middle third fractures of the tibia.

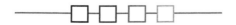

FEATURED ARTICLE

Authors: Sarmiento A, Latta LL.

Title: 450 closed fractures of the distal third of the tibia treated with a functional brace.

Journal Information: *Clin Orthop Relat Res.* 2004;428:261–271.

Study Design: Retrospective Review

▸ 450 closed distal third diaphyseal tibial fractures treated with a functional brace.

Results

▸ 90.0% healed with less than 8 degrees angular deformity in either the frontal or sagittal planes.

▸ 67.1% healed with less than 5 degrees deformity in any plane.

▸ Average final shortening: 5.1 mm (0 to 25 mm).

▸ Final shortening was essentially unchanged from initial shortening at the time of injury.

▸ Overall, 87% healed with shortening less than 12 mm and angulation in any plane less than 8 degrees.

▸ 4 (0.9%) patients developed nonunion.

▸ Average time to union: 16.6 weeks (10 to 40 weeks).

Conclusions

▸ Functional braces for treatment of closed distal third tibia fractures is a viable approach that offers satisfactory clinical and radiographic results in a high percentage of instances.

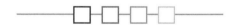

FEATURED ARTICLE

Authors: Martinez A, Sarmiento A, Latta LL.

Title: Closed fractures of the proximal tibia treated with a functional brace.

Journal Information: *Clin Orthop Relat Res.* 2003;417:293–302.

Study Design: Retrospective Review

▸ 108 closed proximal third tibial fractures treated with a functional brace.

Results

▸ Average time to union: 17 weeks (6.6 to 40.5 weeks).

▸ 88% healed with less than 6 degrees angular deformity.

▸ Frontal plane deformities

  ▷ 44% had no angulation in frontal plane

  ▷ 21% had valgus angulation averaging 3.9 degrees (0 to 11 degrees)

  ▷ 35% had varus angulation averaging 5.6 degrees (0 to 15 degrees)

  ▷ 12.3% had angulation greater than 6 degrees (most were varus deformities)

▸ Sagittal plane deformities

  ▷ 55% had no angulation in the sagittal plane

  ▷ 16% had recurvatum averaging 4.6 degrees (0 to 10 degrees)

  ▷ 29% had antecurvatum averaging 4.5 degrees (0 to 11 degrees)

▸ Average final shortening: 3.6 mm (0 to 20 mm).

▸ 3 patients (2.8%) failed brace treatment and underwent surgery.

Conclusions

▸ Functional braces for treatment of closed proximal third tibia fractures is a viable approach that offers satisfactory clinical and radiographic results in a high percentage of instances.

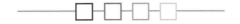

FEATURED ARTICLE

Authors: Bhandari M, Tornetta P III, Sprague S, et al.

Title: Predictors of reoperation following operative management of fractures of the tibial shaft.

Journal Information: *J Orthop Trauma*. 2003;17(5):353–361.

Study Design: Retrospective Observational Study of Patients With Tibial Shaft Fractures Treated Operatively

- Reviewed 200 patients at 2 university-affiliated centers.
- 96% (192/200) had 1-year follow-up information.
- Average age: 38 years, 140 males, 52 females.
- Fracture treatment
  - 42% (80 cases) IM nail
  - 56% (108 cases) plate fixation
  - 2% (4 cases) external fixation
- Fracture classification
  - 60% (115 cases) closed fractures
  - 40% (77 cases) open fractures
    - 19 type I open
    - 34 type II open
    - 13 type IIIA open
    - 11 type IIIB open
- Study's aim was to determine which prognostic factors were associated with an increased risk of reoperation following operative treatment of tibial shaft fractures.
- Assessed 20 different possible prognostic variables.
- Reoperations were defined as any surgery 1 year or less after the initial surgery that was aimed specifically at achieving fracture union
  - Bone grafts
  - Implant exchanges
  - Débridement for infections

Results

- 3 variables predicted reoperation
  - Presence of an open fracture
    - Relative risk of reoperation 4.32, 95% confidence interval (CI) 1.76 to 11.26
  - Lack of cortical continuity ($\leq 50\%$) between the fracture ends following fixation
    - Relative risk of reoperation 8.33, 95% CI 3.03 to 25.0
  - Presence of a transverse fracture
    - Relative risk of reoperation 20.0, 95% CI 4.34 to 142.86

Conclusions

- 3 simple prognostic variables (open fracture, transverse fracture, and postop fracture gap) can assist surgeons in predicting reoperation following operative treatment of tibial shaft fractures.
- Surgeons should avoid distraction at the fracture site (the one variable that is under the surgeon's control) whenever possible in the treatment of tibial shaft fractures.

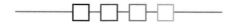

STUDY TO PROSPECTIVELY EVALUATE REAMED INTRAMEDULLARY NAILS IN PATIENTS WITH TIBIAL FRACTURES

Authors: Study to Prospectively Evaluate Reamed Intramedullary Nails in Patients with Tibial Fractures Investigators; Bhandari M, Guyatt G, Tornetta P III.

Title: Randomized trial of reamed and unreamed intramedullary nailing of tibial shaft fractures.

Journal Information: *J Bone Joint Surg Am.* 2008;90(12): 2567–2578.

Study Design: Prospective, Multicenter, Blinded, Randomized Trial

- 1319 adults with tibial shaft fractures
  - ▷ Randomized to treatment with reamed or unreamed IM nail
- Reoperations for nonunion before 6 months were not allowed.
- Primary composite outcome measured at 12 months included the following:
  - ▷ Bone grafting, implant exchange, and dynamization in patients with a fracture gap of < 1 cm
  - ▷ Infection and fasciotomy were considered as part of the composite outcome, irrespective of the postop gap

Results

▸ 1226 patients (93%) completed 1-year follow-up
  ▷ 622 reamed IM nails
  ▷ 604 unreamed IM nails
▸ Overall, 57 (4.6%) required implant exchange or bone grafting for nonunion.
▸ Primary outcome events
  ▷ 105 in reamed group
  ▷ 114 in undreamed group
▸ 826 closed fractures
  ▷ Significantly fewer primary outcome events in reamed group ($P = .03$)
  ▷ This difference was largely due to differences in dynamization
  ▷ 45 primary outcome events (11%) in 416 closed fractures with reamed nails
  ▷ 68 primary outcome events (17%) in 410 closed fractures with unreamed nails
▸ 400 open fractures
  ▷ No significant difference in primary outcome events ($P = .16$)
  ▷ 60 primary outcome events (29%) in 206 open fractures with reamed nails
  ▷ 46 primary outcome events (24%) in 194 open fractures with unreamed nails

Conclusions

▸ This study demonstrates a possible benefit for reamed IM nailing in patients with closed fractures.
▸ This trial demonstrated a substantially lower reoperation rate compared to that reported in previous studies, leading the investigators to conclude that delaying reoperation for nonunion for at least 6 months (part of their postop protocol) may substantially decrease the need for reoperation.

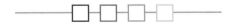

FEATURED ARTICLE

Authors: Whittle AP, Russell TA, Taylor JC, Lavelle DG.

Title: Treatment of open fractures of the tibial shaft with the use of interlocking nailing without reaming.

Journal Information: *J Bone Joint Surg Am.* 1992;74(8):1162–1171.

Study Design: Retrospective Review

▸ 50 open tibial shaft fractures treated with débridement and interlocked unreamed tibial nails.

▸ Average follow-up: 12 months.

▸ Open fracture classification

▷ 3 (6%) grade I

▷ 13 (26%) grade II

▷ 34 (68%) grade III

Results

▸ 48 (96%) united at an average of 7 months.

▸ No malunions.

▸ 4 (8%) infections, all in grade III injuries.

▸ Locking screws broke in 5 patients (10%) but did not result in loss of reduction.

▸ Nails broke in 3 patients (6%).

Conclusions

▸ Prior to the time of this publication, most open tibial fractures were treated either by external fixation, cast immobilization, or an unlocked IM nail (Lottes or Enders nail). The authors concluded that results of the use of an unreamed interlocked tibial nail were comparable to, or better than, other forms of open tibia treatment, including cast immobilization, unlocked IM nailing, and external fixation.

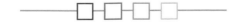

FEATURED ARTICLE

Authors: Bosse MJ, MacKenzie EJ, Kellam JF, et al.

Title: An analysis of outcomes of reconstruction or amputation after leg-threatening injuries.

Journal Information: *N Engl J Med.* 2002;347(24):1924–1931.

Study Design: Prospective, Multicenter (8 Level I Trauma Centers), Observational Study to Determine the Functional Outcomes of 545 Patients With Severe Leg Injuries Resulting in Reconstruction or Amputation

▶ All sustained high-energy trauma below the distal femur defined as the following:

▷ Complicated fractures (Gustilo-Anderson type IIIB and IIIC fractures and selected type IIIA fractures)

▷ Dysvascular limbs (knee dislocations, closed fractures of the tibia, or penetrating wounds with vascular injury)

▷ Major soft-tissue injuries (degloving or severe crush or avulsion injury)

▷ Severe foot and ankle injuries (Gustilo-Anderson type IIIB ankle fractures, all type III intra-articular fractures of the distal tibia and severe hind or midfoot injuries)

▶ 161 patients underwent amputation

▷ 149 underwent amputation during the initial hospitalization (including 37 traumatic amputations)

▷ 12 underwent amputation by 3 months

▷ 6 additional patients underwent amputation by 6 months

▶ The others underwent limb salvage with reconstruction.

▶ Follow-up

▷ 92.1% (502/545) were evaluated at 3 months

▷ 92.3% (503/545) were evaluated at 6 months

▷ 90.5% (493/545) were evaluated at 12 months

▷ 84.4% (460/545) were evaluated at 24 months

- Principal outcome measure was the Sickness Impact Profile
  - ▷ A multidimensional measure of self-reported health status
  - ▷ Scores range from 0 to 100
  - ▷ Scores for the general population average 2 to 3
  - ▷ Scores greater than 10 represent severe disability
- Secondary outcomes included limb status and the presence or absence of major complications resulting in rehospitalization.

Results

- There was no significant difference in the Sickness Impact Profile at 2 years (P = .53)
  - ▷ 12.6 in patients who underwent amputation
  - ▷ 11.8 in patients who underwent limb salvage
- After adjustment for the characteristics of the patients and their injuries, patients who underwent amputation had functional outcomes that were similar to those of patients who underwent reconstruction.
- Predictors of a poorer score for the Sickness Impact Profile included the following:
  - ▷ Rehospitalization for a major complication
  - ▷ Low educational level
  - ▷ Non-Caucasian race
  - ▷ Poverty
  - ▷ Lack of private health insurance
  - ▷ Poor social-support network
  - ▷ Low self-efficacy (the patient's confidence in being able to resume life activities)
  - ▷ Smoking
  - ▷ Involvement in disability-compensation litigation
- Patients who underwent reconstruction were significantly more likely to be rehospitalized (P = .002)
  - ▷ 47.6% in patients who underwent limb salvage
  - ▷ 33.9% in patients who underwent amputation
- Similar numbers of patients returned to work by 2 years
  - ▷ 49.4% in patients who underwent limb salvage
  - ▷ 53% in patients who underwent amputation

Conclusions

▶ Patients with limbs at high risk for amputation can be advised that reconstruction typically results in 2-year outcomes equivalent to those of amputation.

Commentary

▶ This article is one of many published by the Lower Extremity Assessment Project (LEAP) group, which has examined numerous issues surrounding lower extremity limb salvage and lower extremity amputation.

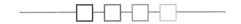

FEATURED ARTICLE

Authors: Vallier HA, Cureton BA, Patterson BM.

Title: Randomized, prospective comparison of plate versus intramedullary nail fixation for distal tibia shaft fractures.

Journal Information: *J Orthop Trauma.* 2011;25(12):736–741.

Study Design: Prospective, Randomized Study

▶ 104 skeletally mature patients with extra-articular distal tibia shaft fractures
  ▷ 56 patients randomized to IM nail
  ▷ 48 patients randomized to large fragment medial plate
▶ Average age: 38 years (18 to 95 years).
▶ The majority were high-energy injuries.
▶ 40/104 (39%) were open injuries.
▶ 28/104 (27%) had ORIF of concomitant fibula fractures.
▶ Ideal treatment of distal tibial shaft fractures is debated
  ▷ Malalignment has been frequently reported after IM nailing of distal tibia fractures

▷ Several studies have reported on knee pain following IM nailing

▷ Plate fixation studies have shown an increased risk of infection and nonunion

▶ Outcome measurements

　▷ Malunion

　▷ Nonunion

　▷ Infection

　▷ Secondary operations

Results

▶ 5.8% (6/104) deep infection rate

　▷ Equal number in both groups

　▷ 5/6 (83%) of infections occurred in open fractures ($P < .001$)

▶ No significant difference in nonunion rate ($P = .25$)

　▷ 7.1% (4/56) nonunion rate in IM nail group

　▷ 4.2% (2/48) nonunion rate in plate group

　▷ There was a trend for nonunion formation in patients who had distal fibula fixation (12% versus 4.1%, $P = .09$)

　▷ All nonunions occurred in open fractures ($P = .0007$)

　▷ 100% of closed fractures united

▶ Significantly more postop angular malalignments of 5 degrees or more in IM nail group ($P = .02$)

　▷ 23% (13/56) in IM nail group

　▷ 8.3% (4/448) in plate group

　▷ 6 additional patients developed malalignment after weightbearing against medical advice

　▷ Valgus was the most common deformity (seen in 16 patients)

　▷ Malunion was more common after open fracture (55%, $P = .04$)

　▷ 85% of patients with malalignment after nailing did not have fibula fixation

▶ No significant difference in secondary procedures

　▷ 11/48 (23%) patients in the plate group underwent 15 secondary procedures

　　≫ 5 were for removal of prominent hardware

　▷ 10/56 (18%) patients in the IM nail group underwent 14 secondary procedures

　　≫ 5 were for removal of prominent hardware

Conclusions

▸ Both nonlocked plating and reamed IM nailing have high primary union rates in distal tibial shaft fractures.

▸ The rates of infection, nonunion, and secondary procedures are similar.

▸ Open fractures have a higher rate of infection, nonunion, and malunion.

▸ IM nailing was associated with more malalignment.

▸ Fibula fixation may facilitate better reduction of the tibia at the time of surgery, but further study is warranted to assess its effect on tibia fracture healing.

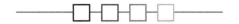

FEATURED ARTICLE

Authors: Koval KJ, Clapper MF, Brumback RJ, et al.

Title: Complications of reamed intramedullary nailing of the tibia.

Journal Information: *J Orthop Trauma.* 1991;5(2):184–189.

This is one of the top 20 cited papers published in the *Journal of Orthopaedic Trauma,* 1987 to 2007.

Study Design: Retrospective Review

▸ 60 acute tibia fractures (in 56 patients) treated with reamed IM nailing.

▸ Average age: 28 years (14 to 63 years), 38 males, 18 females.

▸ Average IM nailing performed: 10 days after injury (0 to 28 days).

▸ Mechanism of injury

  ▷ 39% motor vehicle accidents

  ▷ 14% motorcycle accidents

  ▷ 36% pedestrians struck by motor vehicles

  ▷ 11% other

▶ Fracture classification
  ▷ 48 closed fractures
  ▷ 12 open fractures
    » 11 type I open
    » 1 type II open
▶ 45 were followed to radiographic union.
▶ Average follow-up: 25 months (10 to 63 months).
▶ Complications were categorized into the following:
  ▷ Intraoperative
  ▷ Early postop
    » Certain complications, such as malalignment, are included as early postop complications, presumably because this is when they were first discovered, but these may be better classified as intraoperative complications
  ▷ Late postop

Results

▶ 10% (6/60) rate of intraoperative complications
  ▷ 4 cases of fracture propagation into the nail insertion site
  ▷ 2 cases of poor proximal interlocking screw purchase
  ▷ These complications did not affect final fracture alignment or clinical result
▶ Early postop complications
  ▷ 4 hematomas at nail insertion site
  ▷ 8 malalignments (> 5 degrees varus or valgus)
  ▷ 30% (18/60) neurologic deficits directly related to the procedure, the majority of which were minor sensory neuropraxias of the peroneal nerve
    » 89% (16/18) of these nerve palsies were transient, resolving within 3 to 6 months
    » 2 patients had persistent nerve deficits at 1-year follow-up
▶ Late postop complications
  ▷ 22% (10/45 fractures followed to union) developed patellar tendinitis
  ▷ 2 nonunions
  ▷ 2 deep infections, both of which resolved after local wound care, fracture union, and subsequent nail removal

Conclusions

▸ Overall, 58% (26/45 tibial fractures available for follow-up) developed some complications

▹ Transient neurologic compromise and patellar tendinitis are common complications

▸ Although most complications did not affect the final clinical result, their prevention could speed patient recovery and improve patient comfort.

▸ Surgeon awareness of these problems will allow improved informed consent and should help minimize the extent of these complications.

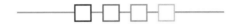

FEATURED ARTICLE

Authors: Bhandari M, Guyatt GH, Tong D, Adili A, Shaughnessy SG.

Title: Reamed versus nonreamed intramedullary nailing of lower extremity long bone fractures: a systematic overview and meta-analysis.

Journal Information: *J Orthop Trauma*. 2000;14(1):2–9.

This is one of the top 20 cited papers published in the *Journal of Orthopaedic Trauma*, 1987 to 2007.

Study Design: Meta-Analysis of Prospective, Randomized Controlled Trials of Tibial and Femur Fractures Treated by Reamed IM Nailing

▸ Authors identified 4 published and 5 unpublished randomized trials that met all eligibility criteria.

▸ Study methodologic quality rating is based on the following:

▹ Randomization and blinding

▹ Population, intervention, and outcomes

▷ Follow-up

▷ Statistical analysis

▸ A 21-point Study Quality Assessment Scale was also used to provide an additional methodologic quality rating.

Results

▸ Nonunion rates ranged from 5% to 33% in different studies.

▸ Pooled relative risk of nonunion in reamed versus nonreamed nails (9 trials, *n* = 646 patients) was 0.33 (95% CI: 0.16 to 0.68; *P* = .004).

▸ Absolute risk difference in nonunion rates with reamed IM nailing was 7% (95% CI: 1% to 11%)

   ▷ One nonunion could be prevented for every 14 patients treated with reamed IM nailing (number needed to treat = 14.28)

▸ Risk ratios for secondary outcome measures

   ▷ Implant failure, 0.30 (95% CI: 0.16 to 0.58; *P* < .001)

   ▷ Malunion, 1.06 (95% CI: 0.32 to 3.57)

   ▷ Pulmonary embolus, 1.10 (95% CI: 0.26 to 4.76)

   ▷ Compartment syndrome, 0.45 (95% CI: 0.13 to 1.56)

   ▷ Infection, 0.98 (95% CI: 0.21 to 4.76)

▸ Sensitivity analyses suggested that reported rates of nonunion and implant failure were higher in studies of lower quality.

▸ Factors that did not significantly affect the relative risk of nonunion between reamed and nonreamed IM nailing

   ▷ Type of long bone fractured (tibia or femur)

   ▷ Degree of soft-tissue injury (open or closed)

   ▷ Whether a study was published or unpublished

Conclusions

▸ Evidence from a pooled analysis of randomized trials indicates that reamed IM nailing of lower extremity long bone fractures significantly reduces rates of nonunion and implant failure compared with unreamed IM nailing.

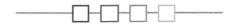

REVIEW ARTICLES

Bedi A, Le TT, Karunakar MA. Surgical treatment of non-articular distal tibia fractures. *J Am Acad Orthop Surg.* 2006;14(7):406–416.

Hiesterman TG, Shafiq BX, Cole PA. Intramedullary nailing of extra-articular proximal tibia fractures. *J Am Acad Orthop Surg.* 2011;19(11):690–700.

Melvin JS, Dombroski DG, Torbert JT, Kovach SJ, Esterhai JL, Mehta S. Open tibial shaft fractures: I. Evaluation and initial wound management. *J Am Acad Orthop Surg.* 2010;18(1):10–19.

Melvin JS, Dombroski DG, Torbert JT, Kovach SJ, Esterhai JL, Mehta S. Open tibial shaft fractures: II. Definitive management and limb salvage. *J Am Acad Orthop Surg.* 2010;18(2):108–117.

Sarmiento A, Latta LL. Functional fracture bracing. *J Am Acad Orthop Surg.* 1999;7(1):66–75.

Tibial Plateau Fractures

chapter 7

FEATURED ARTICLE

Authors: Barei DP, Nork SE, Mills WJ, Henley MB, Benirschke SK.

Title: Complications associated with internal fixation of high-energy bicondylar tibial plateau fractures utilizing a two-incision technique.

Journal Information: *J Orthop Trauma.* 2004;18(10):649–657.

Study Design: Retrospective Review

- 83 bicondylar tibial plateau fractures (AO/OTA type-41-C3) treated with ORIF (dual plating using 2 incisions, anterolateral and posteromedial).
- Average age: 44 years (21 to 88 years), 52 males, 31 females.
- Most were high-energy injuries.
- 11/83 (13.3%) open fractures
  - 1 type II, 7 type III-A, 2 type III-B, 1 type III-C
- 12/83 (14.5%) patients had compartment syndrome and underwent fasciotomy.
- Average time from injury to definitive surgical treatment: 9 days.

Hak DJ.
*Rapid Reference Review in Orthopedic Trauma:
Pivotal Papers Revealed (pp 89-96).*
© 2013 SLACK Incorporated.

- Main outcome measures
  - ▷ Type and incidence of complications
  - ▷ Radiographic assessment of articular reduction and axial alignment

Results

- 7/83 (8.4%) developed deep wound infections
  - ▷ 3 (3.6%) of these had an associated septic arthritis
  - ▷ Clinical resolution of infection occurred after an average of 3.3 additional procedures
  - ▷ Presence of a dysvascular limb requiring vascular reconstruction was statistically associated with a deep wound infection (*P* = .006)
- Secondary procedures for complications
  - ▷ 13 patients required removal of symptomatic hardware
  - ▷ 5 patients required a knee manipulation
  - ▷ 2 patients underwent excision of heterotopic bone to improve knee motion
  - ▷ 1 patient required an equinus contracture release
  - ▷ 1 metadiaphyseal nonunion required nonunion repair
- 16/83 (19.3%) developed a DVT.
- Reduction accuracy
  - ▷ 62% had a satisfactory articular reduction
  - ▷ 91% had a satisfactory coronal alignment
  - ▷ 72% had a satisfactory sagittal alignment
  - ▷ 98% had a satisfactory condylar width

Conclusions

- Comminuted bicondylar tibial plateau fractures can be successfully treated with open reduction and medial and lateral plate fixation using 2 incisions.
- Dysvascular limbs requiring vascular repair are at increased risk for deep sepsis.
- The use of 2 incisions, temporary spanning external fixation, and proper soft-tissue handling may contribute to a lower wound complication rate than previously reported.

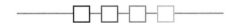

FEATURED ARTICLE

Authors: Barei DP, Nork SE, Mills WJ, Coles CP, Henley MB, Benirschke SK.

Title: Functional outcomes of severe bicondylar tibial plateau fractures treated with dual incisions and medial and lateral plates.

Journal Information: *J Bone Joint Surg Am.* 2006;88(8):1713–1721.

Study Design: Retrospective Review

▸ 83 bicondylar tibial plateau fractures (AO/OTA type-41-C3) treated with medial and lateral plate fixation through 2 exposures.
▸ 31 patients had complete radiographic information
  ▷ Immediate biplanar postop radiographs were evaluated to assess reduction quality
  ▷ Injury radiographs were rank-ordered according to fracture severity
▸ 41 patients completed the Musculoskeletal Function Assessment (MFA) Questionnaire
  ▷ Average age: 46 years, 23 males and 18 females
  ▷ Average follow-up: of 59 months

Results

▸ 2 deep wound infections.
▸ Radiographic review of 31 patients
  ▷ 17 (55%) had a satisfactory articular reduction (≤2-mm step or gap)
  ▷ 28 (90%) had satisfactory coronal plane alignment (medial proximal tibial angle of 87 ± 5 degrees)
  ▷ 21 (68%) had satisfactory sagittal plane alignment (posterior proximal tibial angle of 9 ± 5 degrees)
  ▷ 31 (100%) had satisfactory tibial plateau width (0 to 5 mm)
▸ Patient age was associated with a higher (worse) MFA score ($P = .034$).
▸ Polytrauma was associated with a higher (worse) MFA score ($P = .039$).

▸ Regression analysis demonstrated that a satisfactory articular reduction was significantly associated with a better MFA score (P = .029).

▸ Rank-order fracture severity was also predictive of MFA outcome (P < .001).

▸ No association was identified between rank-order severity and a satisfactory articular reduction (P = .21).

▸ The patients in this series demonstrated significant residual dysfunction (P < .0001), compared with normative data, with the leisure, employment, and movement MFA domains displaying the worst scores.

Conclusions

▸ Medial and lateral plate stabilization of comminuted bicondylar tibial plateau fractures through medial and lateral surgical approaches is a useful treatment method.

▸ Residual dysfunction is common.

▸ Accurate articular reduction was possible in about half of the patients and was associated with better outcomes within the confines of the injury severity.

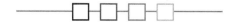

FEATURED ARTICLE

Author: Canadian Orthopaedic Trauma Society.

Title: Open reduction and internal fixation compared with circular fixator application for bicondylar tibial plateau fractures. Results of a multicenter, prospective, randomized clinical trial.

Journal Information: *J Bone Joint Surg Am.* 2006;88(12):2613–2623.

Study Design: Prospective, Multicenter, Randomized Study

- 83 displaced bicondylar tibial plateau fractures (Schatzker V and VI) in 82 patients.
- Randomized to treatment by
  ▷ Standard ORIF: 40 patients
  ▷ Percutaneous and/or limited open fixation and application of a circular fixator: 43 patients
- Outcome measures
  ▷ Physical examination
  ▷ Radiographs
  ▷ Hospital for Special Surgery (HSS) Knee Score
  ▷ Western Ontario and McMaster Universities Osteoarthritis Index (WOMAC)
    » Includes categories for pain, stiffness, and function
  ▷ SF-36
  ▷ Complications
  ▷ Reoperations

Results

- Significantly less intraoperative blood loss in circular external fixation group ($P = .006$)
  ▷ 213 mL in circular external fixation group
  ▷ 544 mL in ORIF group
- Significantly shorter hospital stay in circular external fixation group ($P = .024$)
  ▷ 9.9 days in circular external fixation group
  ▷ 23.4 days in ORIF group
- There was a trend for patients in the circular external fixation group to have superior early outcome in terms of HSS Knee Scores at 6 months ($P = .064$) and the ability to return to preinjury activities at 6 ($P = .031$) and 12 months ($P = .024$).
- These outcomes were not significantly different at 2 years.
- No difference in total arc of knee motion at 2 years.

▶ No difference in WOMAC Scores at 2 years.

▶ SF-36 Scores at 2 years after injury were significantly decreased compared with the controls for both groups (P = .001 for the circular fixator group and P = .014 for the ORIF group).

▶ There was less impairment in the circular fixator group in the bodily pain category (a score of 46) compared with the ORIF group (a score of 35; P = .041).

▶ Complications

▷ Deep infection rate

≫ 7/40 (18%) in ORIF group

▷ Number of unplanned repeat surgeries, and their severity, was greater in the ORIF group (P = .001)

≫ 37 repeat surgeries in ORIF group

≫ 16 repeat surgeries in circular external fixator group

Conclusions

▶ Both techniques provide a satisfactory quality of fracture reduction.

▶ The authors concluded that circular external fixation is an attractive option because it requires a shorter hospital stay, a marginally faster return of function, similar clinical outcomes, and a lower number and severity of complications.

▶ Patients with this injury treated by either method have substantial residual limb-specific and general health deficits at 2 years.

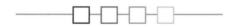

FEATURED ARTICLE

Authors: Weiner LS, Kelley M, Yang E, et al.

Title: The use of combination internal fixation and hybrid external fixation in severe proximal tibia fractures.

Journal Information: *J Orthop Trauma.* 1995;9(3):244–250.

This is one of the top 20 cited papers published in the *Journal of Orthopaedic Trauma,* 1987 to 2007.

Study Design: Prospective Cohort Study

▸ 48 patients with 50 severe proximal tibia fractures treated with limited internal fixation combined with external fixation.

▸ Average age: 39 years (20 to 74 years), 27 males, 21 females.

▸ Average follow-up: 2.7 years (3 to 4 years).

▸ Fracture classification (AO/OTA)

  ▷ 5 A3

  ▷ 6 C1

  ▷ 16 C2

  ▷ 23 C3

▸ Outcome measurements

  ▷ HSS Knee Score

    » 85 to 100 excellent

    » 70 to 84 good

    » 60 to 69 fair

  ▷ Radiographic reduction (joint depression, condylar widening, angulation)

  ▷ Clinical examination

Results

▸ 48 fractures healed following initial procedure.

▸ Average time to union: 12 weeks (8 weeks to 7 months).

▸ 2 nonunions (4%) healed following bone grafting.

▸ 6 (12%) delayed unions (> 3 months).

▸ Average length of time in external fixator: 10 weeks (8 to 14 weeks).

▸ Average knee ROM: 120 degrees (90 to 135 degrees).

▸ Radiographic evaluation

  ▷ 34% (17) excellent results

  ▷ 48% (24) good

  ▷ 12% (6) fair

  ▷ 6% (3) poor

▸ Average HSS Knee Score: 90 (68 to 100)

  ▷ 37 excellent

  ▷ 12 good

  ▷ 1 fair

Conclusions

▶ Combined internal and external fixation is associated with a high percentage of good and excellent results.

▶ It combines the advantages of anatomic, stable fixation with less soft-tissue dissection and eliminates the need for large implants.

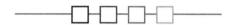

REVIEW ARTICLES
Berkson EM, Virkus WW. High-energy tibial plateau fractures. *J Am Acad Orthop Surg.* 2006;14(1):20–31.
Koval KJ, Helfet DL. Tibial plateau fractures: evaluation and treatment. *J Am Acad Orthop Surg.* 1995;3(2):86–94.

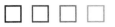

Knee Dislocations

chapter 8

> **CLASSIC ARTICLE**
>
> **Author:** Kennedy JC.
>
> **Title:** Complete dislocation of the knee joint.
>
> **Journal Information:** *J Bone Joint Surg Am.* 1963;45(5):889–904.

Study Design: Retrospective Case Review

- 22 knee dislocations.
- Details injured structures seen in each knee dislocation.
- In addition, reports on experimental cadaveric knee dislocations produced using a stress machine
  - Anterior dislocation produced by knee hyperextension
  - Order of structure injury in anterior dislocation
    - Posterior capsule (occurs at an average of 30 degrees hyperextension)
    - Posterior cruciate ligament
    - Popliteal artery (rupture occurred at an average of 50 degrees hyperextension)
  - Posterior dislocations were harder to create and required greater torques

Hak DJ.
Rapid Reference Review in Orthopedic Trauma:
Pivotal Papers Revealed (pp 97-104).
© 2013 SLACK Incorporated.

Results

- 7 patients had vascular injuries.
- 5 patients underwent above-knee amputation.
- 5 had nerve injuries.
- Repair of collateral and cruciate ligaments was attempted in 6 patients with satisfactory results.
- Many were treated with a course of cast immobilization.

Conclusions

- Complete knee dislocation is an uncommon injury resulting from a variety of mechanisms.
- Associated vascular or nerve injuries occurred in more than 50% of cases.
- Early vascular exploration is mandatory when there is suspicion of a vascular injury.
- Simple treatment of uncomplicated cases may produce surprisingly good results.
- Early repair of major ligamentous injuries results in useful knees.

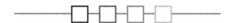

FEATURED ARTICLE

Authors: Twaddle BC, Bidwell TA, Chapman JR.

Title: Knee dislocations: where are the lesions? A prospective evaluation of surgical findings in 63 cases.

Journal Information: *J Orthop Trauma.* 2003;17(3):198–202.

Study Design: Prospective Study

- 63 knee dislocations in 60 patients seen at 2 level I trauma centers over a 5.25-year period.
- Included both knees that were dislocated on presentation and knees that were dislocatable on examination due to severe ligamentous injuries.

▶ All patients with an ankle/brachial index < 0.9 underwent arteriography.

▶ Injured structures were identified on the MRI and at the time of surgery.

▶ Injury mechanism
  ▷ 34 motor vehicle accidents
  ▷ 23 sports injuries
  ▷ 3 falls

▶ All patients underwent open reconstruction within 3 weeks of injury.

Results

▶ Associated injuries
  ▷ 8 had major intra-articular fracture
  ▷ 9 patients (14%) had a popliteal artery injury
    » All had a posterior cruciate ligament (PCL) injury
    » 7/9 had an anterior cruciate ligament (ACL) injury
    » 4 had a sports injury
    » 5 were due to a motor vehicle accident
  ▷ 9 patients (14%) had a peroneal nerve injury
    » All patients with complete peroneal nerve injuries had ACL, PCL, and lateral collateral ligament (LCL) disruptions

▶ Frequency of ligament injury
  ▷ 84% ACL disruption
  ▷ 87% PCL disruption
  ▷ 71% ACL and PCL disruption
  ▷ 44% medial collateral ligament (MCL) disruption
  ▷ 62% LCL disruption

▶ Reattachable ligament avulsions
  ▷ 19% of ACL disruptions had a reattachable ligament avulsion
  ▷ 51% of PCL disruptions had a reattachable ligament avulsion
  ▷ 64% of MCL disruptions had a reattachable ligament avulsion
  ▷ 84% of LCL disruptions had a reattachable ligament avulsion

▶ Common injury patterns
  ▷ Proximal lateral collateral ligament injuries were commonly associated with popliteus tendon avulsions and seldom with distal biceps avulsions
  ▷ Distal LCL injuries were commonly associated with distal biceps avulsions and seldom with popliteus tendon avulsions

▷ Reattachable meniscal capsular avulsions off the tibia occurred predominantly when the collateral ligament injury was a distal avulsion

Conclusions

▸ There is a wide variety of injury patterns in knee dislocations.

▸ Need to have at least 2 ligaments injured to be dislocatable but not necessarily both cruciate ligaments.

▸ Sports injuries have the same pattern of injury as motor vehicle accidents, suggesting similar forces of injury.

▸ There is a high incidence of reattachable avulsion injuries to ligaments and soft tissues in dislocatable knees.

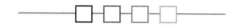

FEATURED ARTICLE
Authors: Harner CD, Waltrip RL, Bennett CH, Francis KA, Cole B, Irrgang JJ.
Title: Surgical management of knee dislocations.
Journal Information: *J Bone Joint Surg Am.* 2004;86-A(2): 262–273.

Study Design: Retrospective Cohort Study

▸ 31 patients with knee dislocations treated by a standard surgical protocol.

▸ Anatomical repair and/or replacement were performed with fresh-frozen allograft tissue.

▸ Excluded from this series were 16 patients treated during the same time period

▷ 4 open knee dislocations

▷ 5 with associated vascular injuries

▷ 3 who were treated in an external fixator

▷ 2 with associated injuries

▷ 2 who were lost to follow-up

▸ 19/31 patients were treated acutely (≤ 3 weeks from injury).

▸ 12/31 patients were treated in a delayed manner (> 3 weeks from injury)

  ▷ Average time of delayed treatment: 6.5 months (5 weeks to 22 months)

▸ Average age: 28 years (16 to 51 years).

▸ Mechanism of injury

  ▷ 17 sports injuries

  ▷ 4 motor vehicle accidents

  ▷ 4 motorcycle accidents

  ▷ 4 work-related accidents

  ▷ 2 falls

▸ Outcome measurements (higher scores = better outcomes for all scores)

  ▷ Lysholm Knee Score

  ▷ Meyers Functional Score

  ▷ Knee Outcome Survey

    » Activities of Daily Living Scale

    » Sports Activity Scale

▸ Average follow-up: 44 months (2 to 6 years).

Results

▸ Average Lysholm Knee Score ($P = .07$)

  ▷ 91 points for acutely reconstructed knees

  ▷ 80 points for knees reconstructed in a delayed fashion

▸ Average Knee Outcome Survey Activities of Daily Living Scale ($P = .07$)

  ▷ 91 points for acutely reconstructed knees

  ▷ 84 points for knees reconstructed in a delayed fashion

▸ Average Knee Outcome Survey Sports Activity Scale ($P = .04$)

  ▷ 89 points for acutely reconstructed knees

  ▷ 69 points for knees reconstructed in a delayed fashion

▸ Meyers functional rating ($P = .14$)

  ▷ 16/19 acutely reconstructed knees had an excellent or good score

    » 7/12 knees reconstructed in a delayed fashion had an excellent or good score

- ROM
  - ▷ Average loss of extension: 1 degree
  - ▷ Average loss of flexion: 12 degrees
  - ▷ No difference between knees reconstructed acutely or in a delayed manner
- 4 acutely reconstructed knees required manipulation because of loss of flexion.
- Laxity tests demonstrated consistently improved stability in all patients, with more predictable results in the acutely treated patients.

Conclusions

- Surgical treatment of knee dislocations provided satisfactory subjective and objective outcomes at 2 to 6 years postop.
- Patients treated acutely had higher subjective scores and better objective restoration of knee stability than did patients treated in a delayed fashion (> 3 weeks after the injury).
- Nearly all patients were able to perform daily activities with few problems.
- The ability of patients to return to high-demand sports and strenuous manual labor was less predictable.

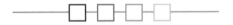

FEATURED ARTICLE
Authors: Stannard JP, Sheils TM, Lopez-Ben RR, McGwin G Jr, Robinson JT, Volgas DA.
Title: Vascular injuries in knee dislocations: the role of physical examination in determining the need for arteriography.
Journal Information: *J Bone Joint Surg Am.* 2004;86-A(5): 910–915.

Study Design: Prospective Study

- 134 acute multiligamentous knee injuries (in 126 consecutive patients) treated over 5.75 years.

- The primary purpose of this study was to evaluate the use of physical examination to determine the need for arteriography in patients with a knee dislocation.
- Results of the physical examination of the vascular status of the extremities were used to determine the need for arteriography.
- Indications for arteriography
  - ▷ Any decrease in pedal pulses, lower extremity color, or temperature
  - ▷ Expanding hematoma about the knee
  - ▷ History of an abnormal physical exam prior to presentation
- All patients underwent serial vascular exams and were admitted to the hospital for at least 48 hours.
- Average follow-up: 19 months (8 to 38 months).
- Physical examination findings, MRI findings, and surgical findings were combined to define the ligamentous damage.

Results

- 9 patients (7%) had flow-limiting popliteal artery damage.
- 10 patients had abnormal physical exam findings
  - ▷ 1 false-positive
  - ▷ 9 true-positive
- Wascher modification of the Schenk knee dislocation (KD) classification
  - ▷ 3 KD-I (multiple ligament injuries that do not include both cruciates)
  - ▷ 1 KD-II (injury of both cruciate ligaments only)
  - ▷ 46 KD-III (injury of both cruciate ligaments and either the posterolateral or posteromedial ligaments)
  - ▷ 45 KD-IV (injury of both cruciate ligaments and both posterolateral and posteromedial ligaments)
  - ▷ 39 KD-V (associated periarticular fracture with multiple ligament injuries)
- Vascular injuries
  - ▷ 1 KD-III
  - ▷ 7 KD-IV
  - ▷ 1 KD-V
  - ▷ The prevalence of vascular injury was highest, 16%, in the KD-IV pattern

Conclusions

▶ Selective arteriography based on serial physical exam is a safe and prudent policy following knee dislocation.

▶ There is a strong correlation between physical exam results and the need for arteriography.

▶ Increased vigilance may be justified in patients with a KD-IV dislocation (dislocation associated with tears of both cruciate ligaments and both posterolateral and posteromedial ligaments) for whom serial exams should continue for at least 48 hours.

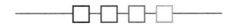

REVIEW ARTICLES

Chhabra A, Cha PS, Rihn JA, et al. Surgical management of knee dislocations: surgical techniques. *J Bone Joint Surg.* 2005;87-A(suppl 1)(pt 1):1–21.

Covey DC. Injuries of the posterolateral corner of the knee. Current concepts review. *J Bone Joint Surg Am.* 2001;83(1):106–118.

Levy BA, Fanelli GC, Whelan DB, et al; Knee Dislocation Study Group. Controversies in the treatment of knee dislocations and multiligament reconstruction. *J Am Acad Orthop Surg.* 2009;17(4):197–206.

Rihn JA, Groff YJ, Harner CD, Cha PS. The acutely dislocated knee: evaluation and management. *J Am Acad Orthop Surg.* 2004;12(5):334–346.

Patella Fractures

chapter 9

FEATURED ARTICLE

Authors: Smith ST, Cramer KE, Karges DE, Watson JT, Moed BR.

Title: Early complications in the operative treatment of patella fractures.

Journal Information: *J Orthop Trauma.* 1997;11:183–187.

Study Design: Retrospective Review

▸ 87 consecutive patella fractures.

▸ A minimum 4-month follow-up was available for 51 fractures

   ▷ 49 were treated with AO modified tension band wiring technique with Kirschner wires (K-wires)

   ▷ 2 were treated with tension band wiring through cannulated screws

   ▷ Postop protocol generally consisted of early knee motion

   ▷ Patients were allowed to bear weight as tolerated in a hinged knee brace locked in extension

Hak DJ.
Rapid Reference Review in Orthopedic Trauma: Pivotal Papers Revealed (pp 105-112).
© 2013 SLACK Incorporated.

Results

▸ Complications
  ▹ 11 fractures (22%) had displacement of ≥2 mm before healing
    » Attributed to technical errors in 5 cases
    » Attributed to patient noncompliance with postop restrictions in 5 cases
  ▹ 2 cases of superficial infection
  ▹ 9 patients with symptomatic hardware required hardware removal

Conclusions

▸ The investigators noted that the incidence of early complications in operatively treated patella fractures is higher than previously reported and that there was a fairly high rate (22%) of fracture displacement ≥2 mm.

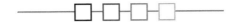

FEATURED ARTICLE

Authors: Carpenter JE, Kasman RA, Patel N, Lee ML, Goldstein SA.

Title: Biomechanical evaluation of current patella fracture fixation techniques.

Journal Information: *J Orthop Trauma.* 1997;11(5):351–356.

Study Design: Cadaveric Study

▸ Examined 3 forms of patellar fracture fixation
  1. Modified tension band (AO technique) with K-wires
  2. 2 parallel 4.5-mm interfragmentary lag screws
  3. Tension band wiring with 4-mm cannulated lag screws
▸ Mechanical testing
  ▹ Amount of interfragmentary separation in simulated knee extension
  ▹ Maximum load to failure at 45 degrees of flexion

Results

▸ Fractures stabilized with a modified tension band were found to displace significantly more than those fixed with screws alone or cannulated screws plus a tension band in simulated knee extensions ($P < .05$).

▸ Fractures fixed with the cannulated screws plus the tension band failed at higher loads (average = 732N) than those stabilized with screws alone (average = 554N, $P = .06$) or those with a modified tension band (average = 395N, $P < .05$).

Conclusions

▸ The investigators concluded that combining interfragmentary cannulated screw fixation with the tension band principle is a simple and reliable method to achieve improved stability of transverse patella fractures.

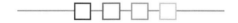

FEATURED ARTICLE

Authors: Saltzman CL, Goulet JA, McClellan RT, Schneider LA, Matthews LS.

Title: Results of treatment of displaced patellar fractures by partial patellectomy.

Journal Information: *J Bone Joint Surg Am.* 1990;72(9):1279–1285.

Study Design: Retrospective Review

▸ 40 patients who underwent partial patellectomy.

▸ These 40 patients were from a cohort of 68 patients who underwent partial patellectomy between 1972 and 1985.

▸ Average follow-up: 8.4 years (1.2 to 18.4 years).

▸ Average age at time of injury: 32 years (11 to 72 years).

- Patients evaluated with a 100-point patellofemoral score
  - ▷ Self-reported findings of knee pain, knee swelling, giving way, movement, and work—45 points
  - ▷ Objective analysis of effusion, ROM, extensor lag, pain, thigh atrophy, and isokinetic quadriceps strength—43 points
  - ▷ Radiographic analysis—12 points
  - ▷ Excellent—score of 90 to 100 points
  - ▷ Good—80 to 89 points
  - ▷ Fair—70 to 79 points
  - ▷ Poor—< 70 points

Results

- Average active ROM: 94% of opposite side.
- Thigh circumference was 100%.
- Quadriceps strength was 85%.
- Overall result
  - ▷ Excellent 20 patients (50%)
  - ▷ Good 11 patients (27%)
  - ▷ Fair 6 patients (15%)
  - ▷ Poor 3 patients (8%)
- There was a significant statistical correlation between the type of fracture and the outcome
  - ▷ The average quadriceps strength in the patients who had had a comminuted fracture was 80% (33% to 120%) compared to patients with transverse fractures whose quadriceps strength was 103% (87% to 139%; $P < .01$)
  - ▷ Average patellofemoral score after a comminuted fracture was 85 points (58 to 99 points) and after a transverse fracture was 93 points (78 to 100 points; $P < .05$)
- 3 patients subsequently had a total patellectomy.

Conclusions

- Partial patellectomy can be an effective treatment for selected patellar fractures.

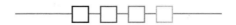

FEATURED ARTICLE

Authors: Marder RA, Swanson TV, Sharkey NA, Duwelius PJ.

Title: Effects of partial patellectomy and reattachment of the patellar tendon on patellofemoral contact areas and pressures.

Journal Information: *J Bone Joint Surg Am.* 1993;75(1):35–45.

Study Design: Cadaveric Study

▶ Examined varying degrees of partial patellectomy and anterior, middle, or posterior attachment of the patellar tendon.

▶ Knee joints were loaded by application of a flexion moment, which was resisted by the extension moment of the quadriceps mechanism.

▶ Patellofemoral contact was measured with the use of pressure-sensitive film, at 30, 60, and 90 degrees of knee flexion.

▶ Inferior partial patellectomy, with sequential removal of 20%, 40%, and 60% of the articular surface, was made with an oscillating saw.

Results

▶ Partial patellectomy, regardless of the position of the tendon reattachment, decreased the patellofemoral contact area and increased contact pressure.

▶ Partial patellectomy altered the pattern of contact, shifting the contact proximally.

▶ With the exception of the 20% patellectomy with anterior reattachment of the patellar tendon, partial patellectomy resulted in significantly decreased contact areas ($P < .05$).

▶ Irrespective of the extent of the patellectomy, anterior reattachment of the patellar tendon produced contact areas most similar to those of the unaltered specimens.

▶ Posterior reattachment was associated with the greatest decrease in contact area for each level of patellectomy, at every angle of flexion ($P < .05$).

▶ After a 60% patellectomy, patellofemoral contact was altered markedly, with the contact area reduced to less than 50% of the control values regardless of the position of the patellar tendon reattachment.

Conclusions

▶ Cadaveric in vitro measurements showed that partial patellectomy is associated with significant changes in patellofemoral contact areas and pressures.

▶ Based on these findings, the authors cannot support the clinical recommendation for treatment of comminuted patellar fractures with excision of comminuted fragments and repair of the patellar tendon to the posterior aspect of the patella.

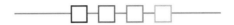

FEATURED ARTICLE

Authors: Sutton FS Jr, Thompson CH, Lipke J, Kettelkamp DB.

Title: The effect of patellectomy on knee function.

Journal Information: *J Bone Joint Surg Am.* 1976;58(4):537–540.

Study Design: Retrospective Cohort Study

▶ 26 complete and 11 partial patellectomies following patellar fracture.

▶ Average follow-up: 63.7 months.

▶ Average age: 42.9 years (22 to 72 years).

Results

▶ Partial patellectomy patients

  ▷ Had less pain with activity and less pain at rest, could squat more easily and walk farther, had fewer problems negotiating stairs and rough ground, and had a higher activity level than patients with a complete patellectomy; however, the differences were not significant

▶ Partial and complete patellectomy caused an equal loss of active and passive ROM.

- Complete patellectomy resulted in greater ligament instability, quadriceps atrophy, and loss of quadriceps strength compared with partial patellectomy
  - ▷ Quadriceps strength in knees with complete patellectomy averaged 62 kg less than normal, a 49% reduction of the strength of the normal extensor mechanism ($P < .001$)
  - ▷ Complete patellectomy caused a reduction in the degree of stance-phase flexion during level walking and negotiating stairs

Conclusions

- Partial patellectomy should be performed instead of complete patellectomy whenever feasible in order to maximize knee stability and function.

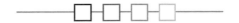

FEATURED ARTICLE

Authors: Lebrun CT, Langford JR, Sagi HC.

Title: Functional outcomes after operatively treated patella fractures.

Journal Information: *J Orthop Trauma.* 2012;26(7):422–426.

Study Design: Prospective Cohort Study

- 40 patients who underwent operative treatment of a displaced patella fracture with a minimum 1-year follow-up
  - ▷ 15 treated with ORIF using tension band wiring with K-wires
  - ▷ 10 treated with ORIF using tension band wiring with cannulated screws
  - ▷ 2 treated with longitudinal anterior banding with cerclage
  - ▷ 13 treated with partial patellectomy
- This cohort was selected from 241 patients who underwent patellar fracture operative treatment over a 16-year period.

- Excluded patients with ipsilateral or contralateral femur and tibial fractures, knee dislocations, spinal cord injury with motor deficit, and medical conditions that severely limited mobility.
- Outcome measurements
  - ▷ SF-36
  - ▷ Knee Injury and Osteoarthritis Outcome Scores
  - ▷ ROM
  - ▷ Strength testing
- Average follow-up: 6.5 years (1.25 to 17 years).

Results

- Average normalized SF-36 and Knee Injury and Osteoarthritis Outcome Scores were statistically different from reference population norms.
- 52% of cases required removal of symptomatic hardware.
- 38% of patients with retained hardware reported hardware-related pain at least some of the time.
- 20% had an extensor lag greater than 5 degrees.
- 38% had > 5 degrees restriction of flexion.
- 15% had > 5 degrees restriction of extension.
- 26% average isometric extension deficit for peak torque.

Conclusions

- Patients have significant symptomatic complaints and functional deficits following patella fracture operative treatment that persist at a average of 6.5 years at follow-up.

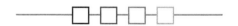

REVIEW ARTICLE
Melvin JS, Mehta S. Patellar fractures in adults. *J Am Acad Orthop Surg.* 2011;19(4):198–207.

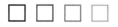

Supracondylar Femur Fractures

chapter 10

FEATURED ARTICLE

Authors: Markmiller M, Konrad G, Sudkamp N.

Title: Femur-LISS and distal femoral nail for fixation of distal femoral fractures: are there differences in outcome and complications?

Journal Information: *Clin Orthop.* 2004;426:252–257.

Study Design: Prospective Cohort Study

▸ 39 patients with distal femur fractures treated with either of the following:
  ▷ Less invasive stabilization system (LISS) (Synthes, Paoli, PA)—20 patients
  ▷ Distal femoral IM nail—19 patients
▸ Outcome measurements
  ▷ Rates of axial deviation
  ▷ Nonunion
  ▷ Infection
  ▷ Lysholm-Gillquist Score
    » Swelling
    » Pain with function (instability)
    » Muscle size

Hak DJ.
*Rapid Reference Review in Orthopedic Trauma:
Pivotal Papers Revealed (pp 113-118).*
© 2013 SLACK Incorporated.

- Average patient age
  - ▷ 57 years (17 to 83) in plate group
  - ▷ 44 years (20 to 77) in IM nail group
- Similar distribution of simple and complex fracture types in the 2 groups.
- CT scans obtained after fracture healing to assess alignment.

Results

- No significant difference in average knee ROM
  - ▷ 110 degrees in plate group
  - ▷ 103 degrees in nail group
- No significant difference in Lysholm-Gillquist Score.
- Nonunion requiring additional surgery
  - ▷ 2/20 in the LISS plate group
  - ▷ 1/19 in the IM nail group
- 1 bone graft procedure for delayed union in IM nail group.
- 1 wound infection in the IM nail group.
- Average time to union (nonunion cases excluded)
  - ▷ 13.8 weeks in the LISS plate group
  - ▷ 15.6 weeks in the IM nail group
- Clinically significant malalignments
  - ▷ 3 malalignments in the plate group
    - » 2 varus > 5 degrees
    - » 1 external rotation deformity > 15 degrees
  - ▷ 2 malalignments in the nail group
    - » 1 varus > 5 degrees
    - » 1 external rotation deformity > 15 degrees

Conclusions

- Both minimally invasive implants had good outcomes for treatment of distal femoral fractures and did not differ significantly in their infection rates, malalignments, and subjective and objective findings at the 1-year follow-up.
- Both were superior to historical outcomes of the dynamic condylar screw/plate in terms of infection and axial malalignment.

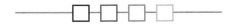

FEATURED ARTICLE

Authors: Kregor PJ, Stannard JA, Zlowodzki M, Cole PA.

Title: Treatment of distal femur fractures using the less invasive stabilization system.

Journal Information: *J Orthop Trauma.* 2004;18(8):509–520.

Study Design: Retrospective Analysis of Prospectively Enrolled Patients Who Sustained a Distal Femur Fracture Treated With the Less Invasive Stabilization System

▸ 3 surgeons at 2 university trauma centers in the United States.

▸ The LISS system was the first locked plate construct available for treatment of distal femur and proximal tibial fractures.

▸ Prior to this treatment, there was a frequent need for bone grafting to achieve union.

▸ 123 distal femur fractures treated in 119 consecutive patients.

▸ 103 fractures in 99 patients were followed until union.

▸ Average follow-up: 14 months (3 to 50 months).

▸ Outcome measurements
  ▷ Perioperative complications
  ▷ Radiographic union
  ▷ Infection rate
  ▷ Loss of fixation
  ▷ Alignment
  ▷ ROM

Results

▸ 93% (96/103) of fractures healed without bone grafting.

▸ 18 patients required secondary surgical procedures
  ▷ 7 subsequently underwent bone grafting and all achieved union

▸ Complications
  ▷ 5 loss of fixation proximally
  ▷ 2 nonunions
  ▷ 3 acute infections
  ▷ 6% (6/103) malreduction

- No loss of fixation distally, despite 30 patients being older than 65 years.
- 11 patients had limited motion, and these patients were characterized by delayed reconstruction due to polytrauma, closed head injury, infection, complex fractures, and extensor mechanism injuries.
- Average knee ROM: 1 to 109 degrees.

Conclusions

- LISS treatment of distal femur fractures results in high union rates without the need for autogenous bone grafting, a low infection rate, and maintenance of distal femoral fixation.

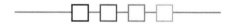

FEATURED ARTICLE

Authors: Bolhofner BR, Carmen B, Clifford P.

Title: The results of open reduction and internal fixation of distal femur fractures using a biologic (indirect) reduction technique.

Journal Information: *J Orthop Trauma*. 1996;10(6):372–377.

Study Design: Retrospective Review

- 57 AO/OTA type A or C supracondylar femur fractures treated by ORIF using indirect reduction techniques by a single surgeon.
- No bone grafting or dual plating was used.
- Average age: 44 years (16 to 88 years), 27 males, 30 females.
- 11 (19%) open fractures
  - 6 type I, 3 type II, 2 type IIIA
- All patients were followed for at least 1 year after injury.
- Surgical technique focused on indirect reduction, rather than using extensive periosteal elevation and direct fracture reduction, in order to preserve the vascular attachments to the bony fragments.
- All patients had use of continuous passive motion postop.

- Functional rating according to modified Schatzker Scale 1 month after full weightbearing and at 1 year
  ▷ Excellent: anatomic alignment, flexion > 120 degrees, < 5 degrees flexion contracture, < 1 cm shortening, minimal pain, no arthritis
  ▷ Good: < 5 degrees varus, flexion 100 to 120 degrees, 5 to 10 degrees flexion contracture, < 1.5 cm shortening, occasional mild discomfort, no arthritis
  ▷ Fair: > 5 degrees varus, flexion 90 to 100 degrees, > 10 degrees flexion contracture, mild to moderate discomfort, radiographic arthritis
  ▷ Poor: < 90 degrees flexion, > 2 cm shortening, nonunion or malunion, severe discomfort, need for ambulatory assistive device

Results

- Average time to union: 10.7 weeks (8 to 16 weeks).
- 2 delayed unions (healing > 16 weeks).
- No hardware failures.
- Modified Schatzker Scale
  ▷ 84% good or excellent
  ▷ 11% fair
  ▷ 5% poor
- Fair and poor results tended to occur in more severe fractures and were primarily due to limited knee motion.
- Multiple regression analysis identified 3 factors related to successful outcome
  1. Patient age (> 67 years had worse outcome; $P < .037$)
  2. Fracture type (C2 and C3 pattern worse than A2, A3, and C1; $P < .002$)
  3. Clinical rating at 1 month postunion related to 1-year result ($P < .001$)
- Complications
  ▷ 2 broken screws
  ▷ 1 deep infection
  ▷ 1 malunion

Conclusions

- Biologic reduction techniques, although they provided excellent bone healing capability, did not guarantee universally satisfactory outcomes.

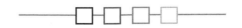

REVIEW ARTICLES

Gwathmey FW Jr, Jones-Quaidoo SM, Kahler D, Hurwitz S, Cui Q. Distal femoral fractures: current concepts. *J Am Acad Orthop Surg.* 2010;18(10):597–607.

Zlowodzki M, Bhandari M, Marek DJ, Cole PA, Kregor PJ. Operative treatment of acute distal femur fractures: systematic review of 2 comparative studies and 45 case series (1989 to 2005). *J Orthop Trauma.* 2006;20(5):366–371.

Femoral Shaft and Subtrochanteric Femur Fractures

11

> **CLASSIC ARTICLE**
>
> **Authors:** Bone LB, Johnson KD, Weigelt J J, Scheinberg R.
>
> **Title:** Early versus delayed stabilization of femoral fractures: a prospective randomized study.
>
> **Journal Information:** *J Bone Joint Surg Am.* 1989;71(3):336–340.

Study Design: Randomized Controlled Trial

- 178 patients with femur fractures randomized to
  - Early stabilization (< 24 hours), *n* = 88
    - 42 patients with isolated femur fractures
    - 46 patients with multiple injuries
  - Delayed stabilization (≥ 48 hours), *n* = 90
    - 53 patients with isolated femur fractures
    - 37 patients with multiple injuries
- Designed to study whether IM nailing with 24 hours of injury would influence the incidence of pulmonary complications.

Results

- Early stabilization decreased pulmonary complications.

Hak DJ.
Rapid Reference Review in Orthopedic Trauma: Pivotal Papers Revealed (pp 119-130).
© 2013 SLACK Incorporated.

- Complication rates
  - ▷ Adult respiratory distress syndrome
    - » 1.1% in early treatment group
    - » 6.7% in delayed treatment group
  - ▷ Pulmonary dysfunction
    - » 0% in early treatment group
    - » 2.2% in delayed treatment group
  - ▷ Fat embolism
    - » 0% in early treatment group
    - » 2.2% in delayed treatment group
  - ▷ Abnormal blood gases
    - » 22% in early treatment group
    - » 50% in delayed treatment group
  - ▷ Pulmonary embolism
    - » 1.1% in early treatment group
    - » 3.3% in delayed treatment group
- Multiply injured patients treated with early stabilization also had decreased hospital stay (17.3 versus 26.6 days).
- Multiply injured patients treated with early stabilization also had decreased intensive care unit stay (2.8 versus 7.6 days).

Conclusions

- The authors provided an overwhelming recommendation that early stabilization of long bone fractures should be performed in multiply injured patients.
- When early stabilization of long bone fractures is done in conjunction with early intubation, ventilatory support, and proper management of fluids, the rate of pulmonary failure in these patients will be drastically reduced and will lead to dramatic savings.

Commentary

- Prior to this landmark study, patients were commonly treated in traction, often leading to deterioration of their condition and even death. While randomized trials are now common, this was rare in orthopedic surgery at the time of the study. The results of this study led to a dramatic shift in the management of trauma patients.

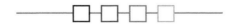

FEATURED ARTICLE

Authors: Winquist RA, Hansen ST Jr, Clawson DK.

Title: Closed intramedullary nailing of femoral fractures: a report of five hundred and twenty cases.

Journal Information: *J Bone Joint Surg Am.* 1984;66(4):529–539.

Study Design: Retrospective Case Series

▸ 500 patients with 520 femoral shaft fractures treated with an IM nail.

▸ Minimum 1-year follow-up in 88.4% of patients.

▸ At the time of the study, there was concern that early IM nailing would lead to fat embolism and so initially IM nailing was delayed for 5 to 7 days, while near the end of the study IM nailing was done immediately.

▸ There was also skepticism that IM nailing of open fractures would lead to a high infection rate.

▸ IM nails used in this study were Kuntscher-style open section nails.

▸ Interlocking was performed for length-unstable fractures.

Results

▸ Mortality rate 2.2% (11 patients)

▷ 1 due to severe brain trauma

▷ 5 due to associated multiple injuries

▷ 3 died in nursing home; average age: 75 years

▷ 2 due to unrelated causes

▸ 87% union rate at 3 months.

▸ Complications

▷ Fat embolism syndrome

▷ External rotation malunion

▷ Peroneal nerve palsy

▷ Shortening

▷ Pulmonary embolism

▷ Valgus angulation

▷ Infection

Conclusions

▸ The authors concluded that IM nailing is an ideal treatment for patients with femoral shaft fractures.

▸ When properly selected, femoral shaft fractures can be treated successfully by IM nailing with minimum complications.

▸ The immediate use of this method demands that the patient be evaluated carefully for associated injuries and be resuscitated adequately.

▸ The authors recommended that primary nailing not be attempted in the multiply injured patient unless an experienced multidisciplinary team is available to manage potential problems.

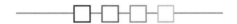

FEATURED ARTICLE

Authors: Nowotarski PJ, Turen CH, Brumback RJ, Scarboro JM.

Title: Conversion of external fixation to intramedullary nailing for fractures of the shaft of the femur in multiply injured patients.

Journal Information: *J Bone Joint Surg Am.* 2000;82(6):781–788.

Study Design: Retrospective Review

▸ 54 multiply injured patients with 59 femoral shaft fractures treated with early external fixation followed by planned conversion to IM nail fixation.

▸ Average age: 33 years (15 to 71 years), 35 males, 19 females.

▸ Average Injury Severity Score: 29 (13 to 43).

▸ Average Glasgow Coma Scale Score: 11 (3 to 15).

▸ 44 patients had additional orthopedic injuries

  ▷ Average additional orthopedic injuries: 3 (0 to 8)

▸ Associated injuries such as severe brain injury, solid-organ rupture, chest trauma, and aortic tears were common.

- Fracture classification
  - ▷ 40 closed fractures
  - ▷ 19 open fractures
    - » 3 type II
    - » 8 type IIIA
    - » 8 type IIIC
- All femur shaft fractures were stabilized with a unilateral external fixator within 24 hours of injury.
- Average follow-up: 12 months (6 to 87 months).

Results

- Average duration of external fixation: 7 days (1 to 49 days).
- 55 fractures were converted from external fixation to IM nail in a one-stage procedure.
- 4 fractures with draining pin sites were treated by external fixator removal followed by skeletal traction to allow pin site healing
  - ▷ Average time in skeletal traction prior to IM nailing: 10 days (8 to 15 days)
- 56/57 (97%) fractures healed within 6 months.
- 3 major complications
  - ▷ 1 patient died from pulmonary embolism prior to fracture union
  - ▷ 1 refractory infected nonunion
  - ▷ 1 nonunion successfully treated with exchange nailing
- 1.7% infection rate.
- 4 minor reoperations
  - ▷ 2 manipulations for knee stiffness
  - ▷ 2 correction of rotational deformity
- Average knee motion: 107 degrees (60 to 140 degrees).

Conclusions

- Immediate external fixation followed by early closed IM nailing is a safe treatment method for fractures of the shaft of the femur in selected multiply injured patients who cannot tolerate IM nailing but who may benefit from long bone fixation.
- While it remains unknown how long external fixation can safely remain in place before there is an increase in infection risk with conversion to IM nailing, many surgeons attempt to convert within 2 weeks.

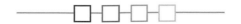

FEATURED ARTICLE

Authors: Ricci WM, Schwappach J, Tucker M, et al.

Title: Trochanteric versus piriformis entry portal for the treatment of femoral shaft fractures.

Journal Information: *J Orthop Trauma.* 2006;20(10):663–667.

Study Design: Prospective, Multicenter (4 Surgeons, 4 Centers) Nonrandomized Cohort Study

- Choice of starting point was at the discretion of the treating surgeon.
- 108 patients treated for a femoral shaft or subtrochanteric fracture with antegrade nailing
  - ▷ 17 patients excluded (4 deaths, 13 lost to follow-up)
- 91 patients in final analysis
  - ▷ 38 treated with a greater trochanteric starting point
  - ▷ 53 treated with a piriformis starting point
- Outcome measures
  - ▷ Operative time
  - ▷ Fluoroscopy time
  - ▷ Fracture alignment
  - ▷ Fracture healing
  - ▷ Complications
  - ▷ Functional outcome based on the lower-extremity measure

Results

- High rate of union after index procedure in both groups
  - ▷ 37/38 greater trochanteric entry site cases healed
  - ▷ 52/53 piriformis entry site cases healed
- 1 malalignment
  - ▷ In greater trochanteric entry site group, 12 degrees external rotation malalignment
- 2 infections, 1 in each group
- No significant difference in average operative time (P = .08)
  - ▷ 75 minutes in piriformis entry group
  - ▷ 62 minutes in greater trochanteric entry group

- Significantly more fluoroscopy time in the piriformis entry group ($P < .05$)
  ▷ 153 seconds in piriformis entry group
  ▷ 95 seconds in greater trochanteric entry group
- In obese patients (body mass index > 30), operative time was 30% greater ($P < .05$), and the fluoroscopy time was 73% higher ($P < .02$) in the piriformis entry group.
- Patients from both groups had a similar initial decline and subsequent improvement in function over time ($P > .05$).

Conclusions

- Trochanteric insertion femoral nails have equally high union rates, equally low complication rates, and functional results similar to conventional antegrade femoral nailing through the piriformis fossa.
- Trochanteric insertion femoral nails have the benefit of decreased fluoroscopy time and decreased operative time in patients who are obese.

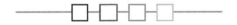

FEATURED ARTICLE

Authors: Bosse MJ, Mackenzie EJ, Riemer BL, et al.

Title: Adult respiratory distress syndrome, pneumonia, and mortality following thoracic injury and a femoral fracture treated either with intramedullary nailing with reaming or with a plate: a comparative study.

Journal Information: *J Bone Joint Surg Am.* 1997;79-A(6):799–809.

Study Design: Retrospective Review

- Multiply injured patients (Injury Severity Score ≥ 17) with femoral shaft fractures and/or thoracic injuries (Abbreviated Injury Scale Score ≥ 2) treated over 12 years.
- Femur fractures at Center I were routinely treated with a reamed IM nail
  ▷ 217/229 (95%) femur fractures treated with reamed IM nail

▶ Femur fractures at Center II were routinely treated with plate fixation

  ▷ 206/224 (92%) femur fractures treated with plate fixation

▶ This difference in routine treatment was used to investigate the effect of acute femoral reaming on the occurrence of acute respiratory distress syndrome (ARDS) in multiply injured patients who had a chest injury.

▶ Investigators evaluated 3 groups of patients

  1. Patients with a femur fracture and thoracic injury

  2. Patients with a femur fracture but no thoracic injury

  3. Patients with a thoracic injury but no femoral or tibial fracture (studied to evaluate whether the 2 centers had a difference in their ARDS rates)

▶ Data collection

  ▷ Requirements for fluid resuscitation were calculated for the first 24 hours

  ▷ Duration of intubation

  ▷ Duration of hospitalization

  ▷ Occurrence of adverse outcomes (death, multiple organ failure, adult respiratory distress syndrome, pneumonia, and pulmonary embolism)

▶ Groups of patients were analyzed by logistic regression to determine if the type of femoral fracture fixation affected the rate of ARDS and mortality

  ▷ Patients analyzed as a whole

  ▷ Patients analyzed after stratifying into subgroups

    ≫ With and without thoracic injury

    ≫ Injury Severity Score < 30 and ≥ 30

Results

▶ Overall occurrence of ARDS in patients with a femur fracture was only 2% (10/453 patients).

▶ No difference between centers in ARDS rates in patients with a thoracic injury only (no associated femur fracture)

  ▷ 6% (8/129 patients) at Center I

  ▷ 8% (10/125 patients) at Center II

- Rate of ARDS in patients with a femur fracture without a thoracic injury did not differ substantially between the 2 treatment groups ($P = .37$)
  ▷ 3% (4/118) in IM nail group
  ▷ 1% (1/114) in plate fixation group
- Rate of ARDS in patients with a femur fracture and a thoracic injury did not differ substantially between the 2 treatment groups ($P > .5$)
  ▷ 3% (3/117) in IM nail group
  ▷ 2% (2/104) in plate fixation group
- Occurrence of pneumonia, pulmonary embolism, failure of multiple organs, or death in patients with a femur fracture and thoracic injury did not differ substantially between the 2 treatment groups
  ▷ Pneumonia ($P = .14$)
    » 7% (8/118) in IM nail group
    » 3% (3/114) in plate fixation group
  ▷ Pulmonary embolism ($P = .49$)
    » 0% in IM nail group
    » 1% (1/114) in plate fixation group
  ▷ Multiple organ failure ($P > .5$)
    » 1% (1/118) in IM nail group
    » 0% in plate fixation group
  ▷ Death ($P > .5$)
    » 3% (3/118) in IM nail group
    » 4% (4/114) in plate fixation group

Conclusions

- The authors concluded that IM nailing with reaming for acute stabilization of femur fractures in multiply injured patients who have a thoracic injury does not increase the occurrence of ARDS, pulmonary embolism, failure of multiple organs, pneumonia, or death.

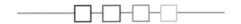

FEATURED ARTICLE

Authors: Lee PC, Hsieh PH, Yu SW, et al.

Title: Biologic plating versus intramedullary nailing for comminuted subtrochanteric fractures in young adults: a prospective, randomized study of 66 cases.

Journal Information: *J Trauma.* 2007;63(6):1283–1291.

Study Design: Prospective, Randomized Study

▶ 66 patients with subtrochanteric femur fractures.

▶ Randomized (based on odd or even medical record numbers) to ORIF with the following:

▷ 32 patients—95 degrees dynamic condylar screw placed in minimally invasive manner

▷ 34 patients—Russell-Taylor reconstruction nail

▶ Average age: 36 years (19 to 54 years), 41 males, 15 females.

▶ Average follow-up: 28 months (24 to 42 months).

▶ Outcome measurements

▷ Clinical evaluation

≫ Walking ability

⟩ Parker and Palmer Mobility Score

⟩ 0 to 9, 0 = complete disability, 9 = no difficulty

≫ Pain

⟩ 1 = no pain

⟩ 2 = mild pain not affecting walking or requiring regular medication

⟩ 3 = moderate pain affecting walking and requiring regular medication

⟩ 4 = severe pain, even at rest, requiring stronger analgesics

≫ Active hip ROM

Results

▶ 97% (64/66) achieved union.

▶ One implant failure in the reconstruction nail group and one delayed union in the dynamic condylar screw group required additional surgery to achieve bone union.

- Average time to union: 15 weeks (12 to 24 weeks).
- Time to union was significantly correlated with patient age ($r = 0.689$).
- Hip pain scores were significantly higher (worse) in the dynamic condylar screw group ($P < .05$)
  - ▷ 1.4 in dynamic condylar screw group
  - ▷ 1.2 in reconstruction nail group
- Significantly shorter fluoroscopic times in dynamic condylar screw group ($P < .05$)
  - ▷ Average: 65.5 seconds in dynamic condylar screw group
  - ▷ Average: 85 seconds in reconstruction nail group
- Significantly reduced blood loss in the dynamic condylar screw group ($P < .05$)
  - ▷ Average blood loss in dynamic condylar screw group: 385 mL
  - ▷ Average blood loss in reconstruction nail group: 543 mL
- Significantly fewer patients required blood transfusion in the dynamic condylar screw group ($P < .05$)
  - ▷ 8 patients in dynamic condylar screw group required a transfusion
  - ▷ 20 patients in reconstruction nail group required a transfusion
- No significant difference between the 2 groups in the Parker and Palmer Mobility Score, hip ROM, time to union, or union rate.

Conclusions

- The authors concluded that the reconstruction nail offered no advantages over biologic plating using a dynamic condylar screw for treatment of subtrochanteric hip fractures in young patients (all patients were < 55 years old).
- Uniformly good results can be obtained with dynamic condylar screw fixation using biologically friendly techniques.

Commentary

- While the dynamic condylar screw is no longer widely used for subtrochanteric or supracondylar femur fractures, this study highlights the benefits of a biologically friendly approach to fracture reduction and fixation.
- The subtrochanteric region of the femur is an area of high stress and traditionally has been a challenge to achieve union prior to implant failure.
- Also, see Bhandari et al (*J Orthop Trauma. 2000*;14:2–9) in Chapter 6.

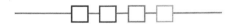

REVIEW ARTICLES

Bedi A, Toan Le T. Subtrochanteric femur fractures. *Orthop Clin North Am.* 2004;35(4):473–483.

Lindsey JD, Krieg JC. Femoral malrotation following intramedullary nail fixation. *J Am Acad Orthop* Surg. 2011;19(1):17–26.

Lundy DW. Subtrochanteric femoral fractures. *J Am Acad Orthop Surg.* 2007;15(11):663–671.

Peljovich AE, Patterson BM. Ipsilateral femoral neck and shaft fractures. *J Am Acad Orthop Surg.* 1998;6(2):106–113.

Ricci WM, Gallagher B, Haidukewych GJ. Intramedullary nailing of femoral shaft fractures: current concepts. *J Am Acad Orthop Surg.* 2009;17(5):296–305.

Intertrochanteric Hip Fractures

CLASSIC ARTICLE

Authors: Baumgaertner MR, Curtin SL, Lindskog DM, Keggi JM.

Title: The value of the tip-apex distance in predicting failure of fixation of peritrochanteric fractures of the hip.

Journal Information: *J Bone Joint Surg Am.* 1995;77(7): 1058-1064.

Study Design: Retrospective Review

- Examined radiographs of 198 intertrochanteric hip fractures (in 193 patients) treated with a sliding hip screw.
- 52 males (27%)
  - ▷ Average age: 71 (20 to 100 years)
- 141 females (73%)
  - ▷ Average age: 79 (19 to 98 years)
- Average follow-up: 13 months (3 to 48 months)
- Fracture classification (Evans as modified by Kyle)
  - ▷ 89 (45%) stable
  - ▷ 109 (55%) unstable
- 19 cases (10%) had fixation failure, with lag screw cutting out of the femoral head in 16 cases (8%).

Hak DJ.
Rapid Reference Review in Orthopedic Trauma: Pivotal Papers Revealed (pp 131-142).
© 2013 SLACK Incorporated.

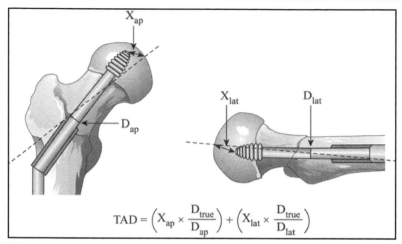

$$TAD = \left(X_{ap} \times \frac{D_{true}}{D_{ap}}\right) + \left(X_{lat} \times \frac{D_{true}}{D_{lat}}\right)$$

Figure 12-1. Technique for calculating the TAD. For clarity, a peripherally placed screw is depicted in the AP view, and a shallowly placed screw is depicted in the lateral (lat) view. (D = known diameter of the lag screw; see text.)

- Examined tip-apex distance (TAD)
  - ▷ Sum of the distance (mm) from the tip of the lag screw to the femoral head apex on the AP and lateral views (Figure 12-1)

Results

- Average TAD in cases with screw cutout: 33 mm (28 to 48 mm).
- Average TAD in cases without screw cutout: 24 mm (9 to 63 mm).
- TAD
  - ▷ < 25 mm no cases of screw cut out
  - ▷ < 30 mm cutout rate 2%
  - ▷ > 30 mm cutout rate 27%
  - ▷ > 35 mm cutout rate 36%
  - ▷ > 45 mm cut out rate 60%
- Multivariate analyses (factors that showed greatest to lowest significance)
  - ▷ TAD > 30 mm (highest significance)
  - ▷ Unstable fracture pattern
  - ▷ Age > 76
  - ▷ Plate angle > 150 degrees (lowest significance)
- In addition to an increased TAD, an increasing age, unstable fracture pattern, and high-angle (150 degrees) side plate were also associated with a significantly increased risk of lag screw cutout.

Conclusions

▸ This simple, reproducible, TAD method is more helpful than previous attempts to describe screw location in the femoral head.

▸ The routine intraoperative estimation of the TAD can increase the surgeon's awareness of the probability of screw cutout and can help guide operative decision making.

▸ Regardless of the zone in which the guide pin is placed, if the proposed position results in a TAD of > 25 mm, the authors recommend reconsideration of the reduction and redirection of the guide pin.

Commentary

▸ In elderly osteoporotic patients, there is limited cancellous bone in the region of the femoral neck. Only near the subchondral bone is there sufficient cancellous bone to achieve lag screw purchase.

▸ Since this paper, surgeons routinely assess the TAD intraoperatively to achieve a TAD < 25 mm in order to decrease the incidence failure due to lag screw cutout.

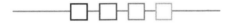

FEATURED ARTICLE

Authors: Kyle RF, Gustilo RB, Premer RF.

Title: Analysis of six hundred and twenty-two intertrochanteric hip fractures.

Journal Information: *J Bone Joint Surg Am.* 1979;61(2):216–221.

Study Design: Paper Includes Both Retrospective and Prospective Reviews of Patients With Intertrochanteric Hip Fractures

▸ Fractures classified by the Evans and Massie classification

▹ Type I: stable, undisplaced

▹ Type II: stable, displaced, varus deformity, fracture of lesser trochanter

▷ Type III: unstable, displaced, fracture of greater trochanter, posterior medial comminution, varus deformity

▷ Type IV: unstable, displaced, comminuted, fracture of greater trochanter, posterior medial comminution with subtrochanteric component

▶ Retrospective review of intertrochanteric fractures treated from 1959 to 1969

▷ 354 were followed to union or longer

▷ 151 were lost to follow-up

▷ Average age: 71 years

▷ 42% males, 58% females

▷ Fracture classification

» 74 (21%) type I

» 127 (36%) type II

» 99 (28%) type III

» 54 (15%) type IV

▷ ORIF with various implants including the following:

» Massie 150 degrees telescoping nail

» Jewett 135 degrees fixed (nontelescoping) nail

▷ Failure rate in stable factures (type I and II): 1.5% (3/201)

▷ Failure rate in unstable fractures (type III and IV): 7.8% (12/153)

▷ Overall mortality rate in first 6 weeks was 11.4%

▷ Overall infection rate was 2.4%

▶ Prospective study that used a sliding Massie nail was used for all type I, II, and III fractures, but they were undecided about what implant to use for type IV fractures

▷ 268 patients followed to union or longer

▷ 59 patients lost to follow-up

▷ Fracture classification

» 57 (21%) type I

» 97 (36%) type II

» 74 (28%) type III

» 40 (15%) type IV

▷ Overall results

» 96% good or excellent

» 1.4% fair

» 2.6% poor

▷ Failure rate in unstable type III fractures was 6.8%

▷ Overall mortality in first 6 weeks was 4.3%

▷ Overall infection rate was 2.1%

▷ Noted that they obtained optimum results when the nail was centered in the femoral head on the AP and lateral views and when the tip penetrated close to subchondral bone (within 1 cm)

▷ Type IV patterns had a higher implant failure rate, except when the Massie sliding nail was used, in which the results were equal to the type III patterns

Conclusions

▶ The Massie telescoping nail proved superior to the Jewitt nontelescoping nail because it allowed a controlled impaction of the fracture fragments to a stable position.

▶ Early ambulation and weightbearing also was a major contributing factor to the improved results seen in the prospective study.

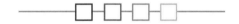

FEATURED ARTICLE

Authors: Haidukewych GJ, Israel TA, Berry DJ.

Title: Reverse obliquity fractures of the intertrochanteric region of the femur.

Journal Information: *J Bone Joint Surg Am.* 2001;83-A(5): 643–650.

Study Design: Retrospective Review

▶ 49 reverse oblique intertrochanteric hip fractures with adequate follow-up who were treated between 1988 and 1998

▷ These cases represented 5% of all intertrochanteric hip fractures during that period

▶ Surgical treatment implants

▷ 16 to 135 degrees sliding hip screw

▷ 15 patients—95 degrees blade plate

▷ 10 patients—95 degrees dynamic condylar screw

▷ 3 patients—cephalomedullary nail

▷ 3 patients—IM hip screw

▷ 2 patients—primary endoprosthetic replacement (not included in results analysis)

▸ 47 ORIF patients were followed until fracture union or revision surgery.

▸ Average clinical follow-up: 18 months (3 to 67 months).

▸ Average radiographic follow-up: 15 months (3 to 60 months).

▸ Results analyzed based on

▷ Fracture pattern

▷ Type of implant

▷ Quality of reduction

▷ Position of implant

▷ Use of bone graft at index operation

▸ Function was assessed based on

▷ Pain

▷ Living situation

▷ Need for walking aids

▷ Need for analgesics

▷ Walking capacity

Results

▸ 15/47 (32%) failed to heal or had failure of fixation.

▸ Failure rate by implant

▷ 9/16 (56%) sliding hip screws failed

▷ 2/15 (13%) 95 degrees blade plates failed

▷ 3/10 (30%) 95 degrees dynamic condylar screws failed

▷ 1/3 (33%) cephalomedullary nails failed

▷ 0/3 IM hip screws failed

▸ Fixed-angle devices (blade plate and dynamic condylar screw) had a significantly lower failure rate than the sliding hip screw ($P = .023$).

▸ Failure rate by reduction accuracy

▷ 11/24 (46%) nonanatomically reduced fractures had treatment failure

▷ 4/23 (17%) anatomically reduced fractures had treatment failure

▷ This difference was not statistically significant ($P = .060$)

▸ Failure rate based on implant position

▷ 11/42 (26%) of ideally placed implants had treatment failure

▷ 4/5 (80%) of nonideally placed implants had treatment failure

▸ 2-year mortality rate of all patients was 33%.

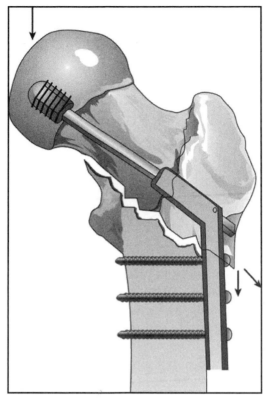

Figure 12-2. Sliding along the fracture plane that can occur when a reverse oblique intertrochanteric hip fracture is treated with a sliding hip screw.

▶ Functional results were poor, with many patients requiring walking aids and losing the ability to walk independently.

Conclusions

▶ Fixed angle devices should be used for reverse oblique intertrochanteric hip fractures.

▶ Loss of reduction and failure occurs with the use of sliding hip screws in this pattern, as shown in Figure 12-2.

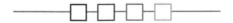

FEATURED ARTICLE

Authors: Sadowski C, Lübbeke A, Saudan M, Riand N, Stern R, Hoffmeyer P.

Title: Treatment of reverse oblique and transverse intertrochanteric fractures with use of an intramedullary nail or a 95 degrees screw-plate: a prospective, randomized study.

Journal Information: *J Bone Joint Surg Am.* 2002;84-A(3): 372–381.

Study Design: Prospective Randomized Study

- 39 elderly patients with reverse oblique intertrochanteric hip fractures
  ▷ 19 patients randomized to treatment with a 95 degrees fixed angle screw plate (Synthes Dynamic [Depuy Synthes, West Chester, PA] condylar screw)
  » Average age: 77 years, 5 males, 14 females
  ▷ 20 patients randomized to treatment with an IM nail (Synthes proximal femoral nail)
  » Average age: 80 years, 7 males, 13 females

Results

- Shorter operative time in IM nail group ($P < .001$)
  ▷ 82 minutes (± 53) in IM nail group
  ▷ 166 minutes (± 48) in 95 degrees screw-plate group
- Fewer blood transfusions in IM nail group
  ▷ 1.45 units (± 1.5) in IM nail group ($P = .006$)
  ▷ 2.95 units (± 1.7) in 95 degrees screw-plate group
  ▷ 11 patients in IM nail group received a transfusion ($P = .008$)
  ▷ 18 patients in 95 degrees screw-plate group received a transfusion
- Shorter hospital stays in IM nail group ($P = .01$)
  ▷ 13 days (± 4) in IM nail group
  ▷ 18 days (± 7) in 95 degrees screw-plate group
- More difficulty, with operative fracture reduction noted in 95 degrees screw-plate group.

- Lower implant failure or nonunion rate in IM nail group ($P = .007$)
  ▷ 1 nonunion in IM nail group
  ▷ 1 nonunion and 6 implant failures in 95 degrees screw-plate group
- More major reoperations in 95 degrees screw-plate group ($P = .008$).

Conclusions

- Investigators recommend the use of an IM implant for treatment of reverse oblique intertrochanteric hip fractures in elderly patients.

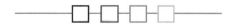

FEATURED ARTICLE

Authors: Bhandari M, Schemitsch E, Jönsson A, Zlowodzki M, Haidukewych GJ.

Title: Gamma nails revisited: gamma nails versus compression hip screws in the management of intertrochanteric fractures of the hip: a meta-analysis.

Journal Information: *J Orthop Trauma*. 2009;23(6):460–464.

Study Design: Meta-Analysis of Randomized Clinical Trials Comparing Gamma Nail With Sliding Hip Screw

- Early clinical trials comparing the Gamma nail (Stryker Orthopaedics, Mahwah, NJ) with a sliding hip screw implant raised concerns about the risk of subsequent femoral shaft fractures in patients treated with first-generation short Gamma nails.
- 25 randomized studies (3464 patients)
  ▷ Separated studies into 3 groups (earlier, recent, and very recent—note some overlap of studies in the different groups)
  ▷ Earlier studies from 1988 to 1996 (1585 patients)
    ≫ Gamma nail treatment increased the risk of femoral shaft fracture 4.5 times compared to sliding hip screw (95% confidence interval: [CI] 1.78 to 11.36, $P = .0014$)

▷ Recent studies from 1997 to 2005 (1879 patients)

    » Gamma nail treatment did not significantly increase the risk of femoral shaft fracture (relative risk = 1.87, 95% CI: 0.73 to 4.82, P = .19).

▷ Very recent studies from 2000 to 2005 (1431 patients)

    » Gamma nail treatment did not significantly increase the risk of femoral shaft fracture (relative risk = 1.65, 95% CI: 0.50 to 5.44, P = .41)

Conclusions

▸ This meta-analysis suggests that prior concerns about increased femoral shaft fracture risk with Gamma nails have been resolved with the newer implant design and improved learning curves with the implant.

▸ Results of earlier randomized trials and meta-analyses should be interpreted with caution in light of more recent evidence.

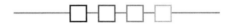

FEATURED ARTICLE

Authors: Palm H, Jacobsen S, Sonne-Holm S, Gebuhr P; Hip Fracture Study Group.

Title: Integrity of the lateral femoral wall in intertrochanteric hip fractures: an important predictor of a reoperation.

Journal Information: *J Bone Joint Surg Am.* 2007;89(3):470–475.

Study Design: Retrospective Review

▸ 214 intertrochanteric hip fractures were treated with a 135-degree sliding hip screw and 4-hole side plate.

▸ All patients were treated at a single hospital and were managed with a specialized hip-fracture protocol designed to optimize surgery, anesthesia, analgesia, postop care, and rehabilitation.

- Patient demographics
  - ▷ Median age: 83 years (23 to 101 years)
  - ▷ 61 males, 153 females

Results

- 25/214 (12%) patients underwent reoperation in the first 6 months postop.
- 15/25 reoperations were due to technical failure
  - ▷ 4 lag screw cutouts
  - ▷ 8 progressive fracture displacements
  - ▷ 3 subsequent fractures around the implant
- 46/214 (21%) had a fracture of the lateral femoral wall.
- The lateral femoral wall is defined as the lateral femoral cortex distal to the vastus ridge.
- 34/46 (74%) lateral femoral wall fractures occurred during the operative procedure and were most frequently occurring during treatment of AO/OTA type 31-A2.2 or A2.3 fractures
  - ▷ Patients with lateral femoral wall fractures had a significantly increased rate of reoperation ($P < .001$)
  - ▷ 10/46 (22%) patients with a lateral femoral wall fracture underwent reoperation
  - ▷ 5/168 (3%) patients without a lateral femoral wall fracture underwent reoperation
  - ▷ Multivariate logistic regression analyses combining demographic and biomechanical parameters indicated that a lateral femoral wall fracture was a significant predictor of reoperation ($P = .01$)

Conclusions

- A postop lateral femoral wall fracture was the main predictor for reoperation after treatment of an intertrochanteric hip fracture with a sliding hip screw.
- Patients with preop or intraoperative lateral femoral wall fractures are not adequately treated with a sliding hip screw.

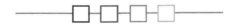

REVIEW ARTICLES

Kaplan K, Miyamoto R, Levine BR, Egol KA, Zuckerman JD. Surgical management of hip fractures: an evidence-based review of the literature. II: intertrochanteric fractures. *J Am Acad Orthop Surg.* 2008;16(11):665–673.

Lindskog DM, Baumgaertner MR. Unstable intertrochanteric hip fractures in the elderly. *J Am Acad Orthop Surg.* 2004;12(3):179–190.

Femoral Head Fractures

chapter **13**

> ### CLASSIC ARTICLE
>
> **Author:** Pipkin G.
>
> **Title:** Treatment of grade IV fracture-dislocation of the hip.
>
> **Journal Information:** *J Bone Joint Surg Am.* 1957;39-A(5):1027–1042.

Study Design: Retrospective Pooled Experience of a Correspondence Club and of Orthopedic Surgeons of Greater Kansas City

▸ 25 femoral head fractures in 24 patients.

▸ Average age: approximately 41 years (20 to 65 years).

▸ Follow-up: 1 year to 18 years.

▸ Data incomplete, with only 7 cases clinically examined by Dr. Pipkin.

▸ Defined the Pipkin classification of femoral head fractures

  ▷ Type I: dislocation with fracture of femoral head caudad to the fovea

  ▷ Type II: dislocation with fracture of femoral head cephalad to the fovea

  ▷ Type III: type 1 or 2 injury associated with a femoral neck fracture

  ▷ Type IV: type 1 or 2 injury associated with an acetabular fracture

▸ Fracture types

  ▷ Type I: 7

  ▷ Type II: 9

Hak DJ.
*Rapid Reference Review in Orthopedic Trauma:
Pivotal Papers Revealed (pp 143-150).*
© 2013 SLACK Incorporated.

▷ Type III: 4

▷ Type IV: 3

▷ Unclassified: 2

▶ Treatment

  ▷ 10 closed reduction

  ▷ 7 open reduction

  ▷ 6 ORIF

  ▷ 2 prosthetic replacements

▶ Outcome grading

  ▷ Good: painless hip, can tolerate weightbearing, and has only a few degrees of motion limitation

  ▷ Serviceable: able to tolerate weightbearing but are still under observation because of incongruity, or hips in which successful salvage procedures have been done

  ▷ Failures: all others

Results

▶ 9 good.

▶ 3 fair (not defined in their article).

▶ 12 serviceable.

▶ 1 death due to multiple injuries.

Conclusions

▶ The best results in this series were achieved by prompt closed reduction followed by traction or immobilization. When this method of treatment was used, bone union of the fracture of the femoral head resulted.

▶ In the cases in which closed reduction could not be successfully done, a small percentage of good results was obtained by open reduction with or without internal fixation.

▶ Open reduction after excision of a blocking or comminuted fragment usually resulted in a hip that could tolerate weightbearing for several years.

▶ Salvage procedures are indicated for hips in which there is irreparable immediate damage and for hips in which there is progressive degeneration.

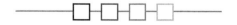

| FEATURED ARTICLE |

Authors: Swiontkowski MF, Thorpe M, Seiler JG, Hansen ST.

Title: Operative management of displaced femoral head fractures: case-matched comparison of anterior versus posterior approaches for Pipkin I and Pipkin II fractures.

Journal Information: *J Orthop Trauma.* 1992;6(4):437–442.

Study Design: Retrospective Review

▶ 26 Pipkin I and II fractures managed operatively over a 15-year period at 2 institutions.

▶ 24/26 had > 2-year follow-up

  ▷ 12 were managed with a posterior surgical approach

  ▷ 12 were managed with an anterior surgical approach

▶ Authors also reported on 17 additional femoral head fractures, including Pipkin III and IV fractures and those without follow-up.

▶ Some authors had indicated that an anterior approach following a posterior hip dislocation is contraindicated because of concerns regarding further damage to uninjured blood supply.

▶ However, anatomic studies have shown that there is minimal, if any, blood supply from the anterior capsule (Trueta J, Harrison MH. The normal vascular anatomy of the femoral head in adult man. *J Bone Joint Surg Br.* 1953;35-B[3]:442–461).

▶ Based on these anatomic data, the authors hypothesized that the anterior approach would have no negative effects in terms of osteonecrosis.

▶ Evaluated

  ▷ Operative time

  ▷ Estimated blood loss

  ▷ Functional results

    ≫ Excellent: ≥ 130 degrees flexion, no pain

    ≫ Good: 90 to 130 degrees hip flexion, minimal pain (functionally insignificant)

    ≫ Fair: < 90 degrees hip flexion, significant pain

  ▷ Radiographic review for reduction accuracy, avasular necrosis (AVN), heterotopic ossification

Results

- ▸ Significantly shorter average operative time in anterior approach group ($P < .05$)
  - ▷ Posterior approach: 4.1 hours
  - ▷ Anterior approach: 2.9 hours
- ▸ Significantly lower average estimated blood loss in anterior approach group ($P < .05$)
  - ▷ Posterior approach: 895 mL
  - ▷ Anterior approach: 430 mL
- ▸ Reductions were within 2 mm in all cases
  - ▷ 1 case in posterior approach group—screws did not engage the fragment
  - ▷ 3 cases in posterior approach group were treated with fragment excision because the surgeon could not adequately view the femoral head fragment
  - ▷ 1 additional case in posterior approach group required an anterior approach for fragment excision
- ▸ Heterotopic ossification (HO)
  - ▷ 3 patients in posterior group developed HO
    - » Average Brooker stage: 2.6
  - ▷ 7 patients in anterior group developed HO
    - » Average Brooker stage: 1.8
    - » 3 patients had less than 100 degrees of hip motion, 1 who underwent HO excision
- ▸ Functional outcomes were identical in the 2 groups
  - ▷ Posterior approach
    - » 8 good or excellent
    - » 4 fair
  - ▷ Anterior approach
    - » 8 good or excellent
    - » 4 fair
- ▸ Radiographic outcomes
  - ▷ Posterior approach
    - » 2 with AVN
    - » 2 with early degenerative arthritis
  - ▷ Anterior approach
    - » No cases of AVN

Conclusions

▸ Because of the greater ease of access of the fracture, the anterior approach is recommended for Pipkin I and II fractures requiring ORIF.

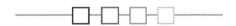

FEATURED ARTICLE

Authors: Stannard JP, Harris HW, Volgas DA, Alonso JE.

Title: Functional outcome of patients with femoral head fractures associated with hip dislocations.

Journal Information: *Clin Orthop Relat Res.* 2000;377:44–56.

Study Design: Retrospective Review

▸ 22 patients undergoing femoral head fracture ORIF.

▸ Average age: 37 years (17 to 72 years), 16 males, 10 females.

▸ Outcome measurements
  ▷ SF-12 (available on only 17 patients)
  ▷ Radiographs
  ▷ Clinical examination

▸ Average follow-up: 24 months (6 to 51 months).

▸ ORIF performed in 12 cases (55%) using a variety of implants
  ▷ Herbert screws (3 cases)
  ▷ Acutrak screws (2 cases)
  ▷ Countersunk 4-mm cancellous screws (2 cases)
  ▷ Cannulated 3-mm screws with threaded washers (5 cases)

▸ Fragment excision performed in remaining 10 cases (45%).

▸ Surgical approach
  ▷ Anterior Smith-Petersen or posterior Kocher-Langenbeck approach or both performed at the discretion of the treating surgeon

Results

▸ Patients whose fractures were stabilized with 3-mm cannulated screws and washers had a poor functional outcome

  ▷ 4 of 5 showed backing out of screws into the joint

▸ 5 patients had evidence of femoral head AVN

  ▷ 4 cases had been treated with a posterior Kocher-Langenbeck approach

  ▷ 1 case had been treated with an anterior Smith-Petersen approach

  ▷ Because of the small number of cases, this was not statistically significant, but odds ratio analysis showed a 3.2 times higher incidence of AVN development when a posterior approach was used

Conclusions

▸ Smith-Petersen anterior surgical approach is recommended for the majority of patients with femoral head fractures.

▸ 3-mm cannulated screws with threaded washers are contraindicated for use in stabilizing femoral head fractures and should not be used in any joint because of dissociation between the screw and the washer.

▸ In terms of prognosis, the Brumback classification system provides superior differentiation of different fracture types compared to the Pipkin classification.

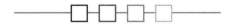

FEATURED ARTICLE

Authors: Henle P, Kloen P, Siebenrock KA.

Title: Femoral head injuries: which treatment strategy can be recommended?

Journal Information: *Injury.* 2007;38(4):478–488.

Study Design: Retrospective Review

▸ 12 femoral head fractures treated from 1998 to 2006.

▸ One patient treated nonoperatively.

- 11 patients treated with ORIF.
- Surgical approach using a "trochanteric flip" (digastric) osteotomy and hip dislocation, allowing inspection of the entire hip joint and accurate fragment reduction under direct visual control.
- Average age: 40 years (29 to 71).
- Average follow-up: 31 months (3 to 96 months).
- Fracture type
  - 1 type I
  - 3 type II
  - 8 type IV
- Outcome assessment
  - Merle d'Aubigne and Postel Score
    - Evaluates hip pain, mobility, and walking
    - 18 points: excellent
    - 15 to 17 points: good
    - 12 to 14 points: fair
    - < 12 points: poor

Results

- 83% (10/12) had good or excellent results.
- 2 patients developed AVN and underwent total hip arthroplasty.
- 5 cases of heterotopic ossification, 4 of which significantly reduced ROM
  - The 2 cases with the most severe HO (Brooker III and IV) had associated closed head injuries

Conclusions

- In comparing their results with earlier published series including their own before changing the treatment protocol, the data suggest a favorable outcome in patients with trochanteric flip (digastric) osteotomy for the treatment of femoral head fractures.
- The authors recommend the trochanteric flip (digastric) osteotomy and hip dislocation for treatment of all larger femoral head fractures requiring ORIF.

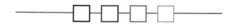

REVIEW ARTICLES

Droll KP, Broekhuyse H, O'Brien P. Fracture of the femoral head. *J Am Acad Orthop Surg.* 2007;15(12):716–727.

Giannoudis PV, Kontakis G, Christoforakis Z, Akula M, Tosounidis T, Koutras C. Management, complications and clinical results of femoral head fractures. *Injury.* 2009;40(12):1245–1251.

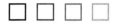

Femoral Neck Fractures

chapter 14

FEATURED ARTICLE

Authors: Haidukewych GJ, Rothwell WS, Jacofsky DJ, Torchia ME, Berry DJ.

Title: Operative treatment of femoral neck fractures in patients between the ages of fifteen and fifty years.

Journal Information: *J Bone Joint Surg Am.* 2004;86-A(8):1711–1716.

Study Design: Retrospective Review

▸ 83 femoral neck fractures in 82 patients between the ages of 15 and 50 years who were treated by ORIF at the Mayo Clinic between 1975 and 2000.

▸ 73 fractures were followed to union, until conversion to total hip arthroplasty (THA), or for a minimum of 2 years.

▸ Average follow-up: 6.6 years (3 months to 23 years).

▸ Fracture pattern
  ▷ 51 displaced
  ▷ 22 nondisplaced

▸ Evaluated effect of various factors on outcome
  ▷ Fracture displacement
  ▷ Reduction quality
  ▷ Capsular decompression

Hak DJ.
Rapid Reference Review in Orthopedic Trauma: Pivotal Papers Revealed (pp 151-164).
© 2013 SLACK Incorporated.

Results

- ▶ 53 fractures (73%) healed with no evidence of osteonecrosis.
- ▶ 17 fractures (23%) developed osteonecrosis
  - ▷ Osteonecrosis developed in 14/51 (27%) displaced fractures
  - ▷ Osteonecrosis developed in 3/22 (14%) nondisplaced fractures
  - ▷ There was a strong trend for displaced fractures to demonstrate a higher rate of osteonecrosis development, but the difference was not significant ($P = .17$)
- ▶ 6 fractures (8%) developed nonunion
  - ▷ 4 nonunions later healed following a second procedure
  - ▷ Nonunion developed in 5/51 (10%) displaced fractures
  - ▷ Nonunion developed in 1/22 (4.5%) nondisplaced fractures
- ▶ Influence of reduction accuracy on outcome
  - ▷ 11/46 (24%) cases with good-to-excellent reduction developed osteonecrosis
  - ▷ 3/5 (60%) cases with fair-to-poor reduction developed osteonecrosis (2 of these also developed a nonunion)
  - ▷ 2/46 (4%) cases with good-to-excellent reduction developed nonunion
  - ▷ 3/5 (60%) cases with fair-to-poor reduction developed osteonecrosis
  - ▷ Only 1/5 cases with fair to poor reduction healed without complication
- ▶ Influence of capsulotomy on outcome
  - ▷ No statistical effect of capsulotomy on development of osteonecrosis ($P = .50$)
  - ▷ 14 displaced fractures underwent open reduction, with direct visualization and therefore had a capsulotomy performed
  - ▷ 4 displaced fractures treated successfully by closed reduction were treated with a capsulotomy
  - ▷ 3 nondisplaced fractures were treated with a capsulotomy, and 1 with aspiration
  - ▷ 4/22 (18%) cases that underwent capsulotomy/decompression developed osteonecrosis
  - ▷ 13/51 (25%) cases without capsulotomy developed osteonecrosis
- ▶ At the time of final follow-up, 13 fractures (18%) had undergone conversion to THA
  - ▷ 11 due to osteonecrosis
  - ▷ 1 due to nonunion
  - ▷ 1 due to osteonecrosis and nonunion
  - ▷ Average time from injury to THA was 7.3 years (3 months to 15 years)

Conclusions

▸ The 10-year hip survival rate following femoral neck fracture in young patients treated by ORIF was 85%.

▸ Osteonecrosis was the main reason for conversion to THA.

▸ Not all patients with osteonecrosis required further surgery.

▸ Initial fracture displacement and quality of reduction influenced the outcome.

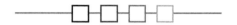

FEATURED ARTICLE

Authors: Gjertsen JE, Vinje T, Engesaeter LB, et al.

Title: Internal screw fixation compared with bipolar hemiarthroplasty for treatment of displaced femoral neck fractures in elderly patients.

Journal Information: *J Bone Joint Surg Am.* 2010;92(3):619–628.

Study Design: Analyzed Data From the Norwegian Hip Fracture Register, Which Is a Prospective Observational Study That Was Initiated in 2005

▸ Compared ORIF versus bipolar hemiarthroplasty for *displaced* femoral neck fractures in elderly patients.

▸ 4335 patients over age 70 with displaced femoral neck fractures
  ▷ 1823 treated with ORIF
  ▷ 2512 treated with bipolar hemiarthroplasty
    » All were contemporary bipolar hemiarthroplasty implants
    » 21% were uncemented hydroxyapatite-coated stems
  ▷ Minimum 12 months follow-up available

▸ Outcomes analyzed included the following:
  ▷ 1-year mortality
  ▷ Number of reoperations

▷ Patient self-assessment of pain, satisfaction, and quality of life at 4 and 12 months

» 12 month questionnaires available for

⟩ 403 treated with ORIF

⟩ 628 treated with hemiarthroplasty

▷ Euro quality of life-5 dimensions (EQ-5D standardized nondisease specific instrument for evaluating health-related quality of life) and EQ-VAS (a 20-cm VAS Health Scale)

Results

▸ 1-year mortality: no significant difference ($P = .76$)

▷ 27% 1-year mortality in ORIF group

▷ 25% 1-year mortality in bipolar hemiarthroplasty group

▸ Number of reoperations

▷ 412 (23%) reoperations in ORIF group

▷ 72 (3%) reoperations in bipolar hemiarthroplasty group

▸ Patient self-assessment at 1 year

▷ ORIF group reported significantly more pain (average of 29.9 versus 19.2, $P < .001$)

▷ ORIF group reported significantly higher dissatisfaction (average of 38.9 versus 25.7, $P < .001$)

▷ ORIF group reported significantly lower quality of life (average of 0.51 versus 0.60, $P < .001$)

Conclusions

▸ The investigators concluded that displaced femoral neck fractures in elderly patients should be treated with a hemiarthroplasty.

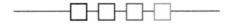

FEATURED ARTICLE

Authors: Lindequist S, Törnkvist H.

Title: Quality of reduction and cortical screw support in femoral neck fractures. An analysis of 72 fractures with a new computerized measuring method.

Journal Information: *J Orthop Trauma.* 1995;9(3):215–221.

Study Design: Retrospective Review

▶ Compared the reduction quality and screw position with the rate of union in femoral neck fractures treated by closed reduction and internal fixation with 2 screws

  ▷ 1 screw placed inferiorly adjacent to posterior femoral neck cortex

  ▷ 1 screw placed posterior adjacent to posterior femoral neck cortex

▶ 75 patients treated

  ▷ 3 excluded (1 deep infection, 1 fall with refracture, 1 bilateral above-knee amputation)

  ▷ 14 patients without known healing complications who died within 1 year were analyzed separately

  ▷ 58 patients followed for up to 2 years or until fracture nonunion made up final study group

    » 13 nondisplaced (Garden I and II)

    » 45 displaced (Garden III and IV)

▶ Radiographs digitally analyzed to quantify accuracy of reduction and position of screws with respect to the femoral neck cortex.

▶ Multivariate logistic regression analysis used to evaluate the initial displacement, reduction quality, cortical support, and different screw positions on the healing rate.

Results

▶ Fracture displacement

  ▷ 100% (13/13) of nondisplaced fractures healed

  ▷ 64% (29/45) of displaced fractures healed ($P < .01$)

▶ Screw position/cortical support

  ▷ There was a significantly higher union rate in displaced fractures in which both screws achieved cortical support compared to those in which only one screw achieved cortical support ($P < .05$)

  ▷ There was a significantly high union rate in displaced fractures in which one screw achieved cortical support compared to those in which neither screw achieved cortical support

  ▷ 16/18 fractures in which both screws were placed within 3 mm of the femoral neck cortex healed

  ▷ 13/22 fractures in which only one screw was placed within 3 mm of the femoral neck cortex healed

  ▷ 0/5 fractures in which neither screws were placed within 3 mm of the femoral neck cortex healed

▶ Reduction quality did not affect the healing rate; however, the number of poorly reduced fractures was only 10%.

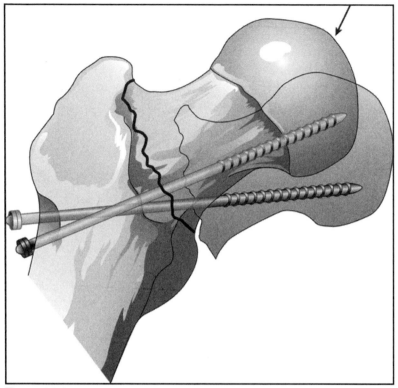

Figure 14-1. When screws are centrally placed in osteoporotic femoral neck fractures, the fracture will typically displace inferiorly until the screw abuts the intact femoral cortex.

Conclusions

▸ The results of this study underline the importance of achieving cortical support for the fixating screws in femoral neck fracture surgery.

Commentary

▸ This paper introduced the importance of cortical support when using screws to fix femoral neck fractures in elderly patients.

▸ Because the cancellous bone in the femoral neck is deficient, femoral neck fractures will typically displace until the screw abuts the intact femoral cortex (Figure 14-1). For optimal results, screws should be placed near the femoral neck cortex, rather than centrally within the osteoporotic femoral neck.

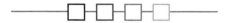

FEATURED ARTICLE

Authors: Bhandari M, Devereaux PJ, Swiontkowski MF, et al.

Title: Internal fixation compared with arthroplasty for displaced fractures of the femoral neck. A meta-analysis.

Journal Information: *J Bone Joint Surg Am.* 2003;85-A(9):1673–1681.

Study Design: Meta-Analysis

▶ Clinical trials that compared internal fixation with arthroplasty for the treatment of displaced femoral neck fractures.

▶ This study's objective was to compare arthroplasty (hemiarthroplasty, bipolar arthroplasty, and total hip arthroplasty) with internal fixation on the following rates:

  ▷ Mortality

  ▷ Need for revision surgery

  ▷ Pain

  ▷ Function

  ▷ Operating time

  ▷ Wound infection in patients with a displaced femoral neck fracture

▶ Identified 14 clinical trials published between 1969 and 2002 that met their eligibility criteria for sound clinical trials.

Results

▶ In terms of reported relative risk, values > 1.0 favor ORIF, while values < 1.0 favor arthroplasty.

▶ Mortality rates

  ▷ 9 trials, with 1162 patients, provided detailed information on mortality rates during the first 4 postop months

  ▷ Mortality rates ranged from 0% to 20%

  ▷ There was a trend toward an increase in the relative risk of death in the first 4 months after arthroplasty compared to internal fixation (relative risk = 1.27)

  ▷ At 1 year, the relative risk of death was 1.04

  ▷ The risk of death after arthroplasty appeared to be higher than that after fixation with a compression screw and side plate but not higher than that after internal fixation with use of screws only (relative risk = 1.75 and 0.86, respectively; $P < .05$)

- Revision surgery
  - ▷ 14 trials with 1901 patients provided data on revision surgery
  - ▷ There was a significantly greater risk of revision surgery following internal fixation (relative risk = 0.23, P = .003)
- Pain relief was similar in patients treated with arthroplasty and in those treated with internal fixation
  - ▷ 6 trials with 1153 patients provided data on pain relief
  - ▷ Pain relief relative risk = 1.12
- Attainment of overall good function was similar in patients treated with arthroplasty and those treated with internal fixation
  - ▷ 12 trials with 1179 patients provided data on patient function
  - ▷ Function relative risk = 0.99
- Infection
  - ▷ 12 trials with 1822 patients provided data on infection
  - ▷ Infection rates ranged from 0% to 18%
  - ▷ Arthroplasty significantly increased the risk of infection (relative risk = 1.81; P = .009)
- Blood loss
  - ▷ 4 trials with 343 patients provided data on estimated blood loss
  - ▷ Patients who underwent arthroplasty had greater blood loss
  - ▷ Weighted average difference: 176 mL
- Operative time
  - ▷ 5 trials with 447 patients provided data on operative time
  - ▷ Patients who underwent arthroplasty had longer operative times
  - ▷ Weighted average difference: 29 minutes

Conclusions

- Treatment of displaced femoral neck fractures by arthroplasty significantly reduces the risk of revision surgery, at the cost of greater infection rates, blood loss, and operative time and possibly an increase in early mortality rates.
- Larger trials are necessary to resolve the critical question of the impact of treatment choice on the early mortality rate.

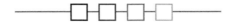

FEATURED ARTICLE
Authors: Taylor F, Wright M, Zhu M.
Title: Hemiarthroplasty of the hip with and without cement: a randomized clinical trial.
Journal Information: *J Bone Joint Surg Am.* 2012;94(7):577–583.

Study Design: Prospective Randomized Study

- 160 elderly patients (age > 70) with displaced femoral neck fractures undergoing hemiarthroplasty.
- Randomized by computer-generated, sequentially numbered, sealed and opaque envelopes
  ▷ Cemented hemiarthroplasty (80 patients)
  ▷ Uncemented hemiarthroplasty (80 patients)
- Average age: 85 years (70 to 99 years), 50 males, 110 females.
- Outcomes assessed the following:
  ▷ Pain
  ▷ Mortality
  ▷ Mobility
  ▷ Complications
  ▷ Reoperations
  ▷ Timed Up and Go (TUG) Score
  ▷ Short Musculoskeletal Function Assessment (SMFA)
  ▷ Oxford Hip Score

Results

- More complications in the uncemented group
  ▷ 63 complications in the uncemented group
  ▷ 28 complications in the cemented group
- Significantly more cases of subsidence in uncemented group
  ▷ 18 cases of subsidence in the uncemented group
  ▷ 1 case of subsidence in the cemented group
- Significantly more intraoperative or postop fractures in the uncemented group
  ▷ 18 cases in the uncemented group (6 intraoperative, 12 postop)
  ▷ 1 case in the cemented group (1 postop)

- No difference in mortality at any time point.
- No difference in SMFA between the 2 groups.
- Oxford Hip Score was significantly worse in the uncemented group at 6 weeks, and although it was poorer at later follow-up times, those differences were not significant.

Conclusions

- Both cemented and uncemented prostheses provided comparable outcomes in terms of pain.
- There were significantly fewer implant complications with the use of a cemented hemiarthroplasty implant.
- There was a trend toward better function and mobility in patients treated with a cemented hemiarthroplasty.

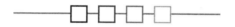

FEATURED ARTICLE

Authors: Keating JF, Grant A, Masson M, Scott NW, Forbes JF.

Title: Randomized comparison of reduction and fixation, bipolar hemiarthroplasty, and total hip arthroplasty: treatment of displaced intracapsular hip fractures in healthy older patients.

Journal Information: *J Bone Joint Surg Am.* 2006;88(2):249-260.

Study Design: Prospective, Randomized, Multicenter Study

- 298 patients with displaced femoral neck fractures.
- Surgeons involved agreed to randomize their patients into either 1 of 3 treatments or 1 of 2 treatments
  - ▷ 3-way randomization
    - » Reduction and internal fixation
    - » Cemented bipolar hemiarthroplasty
    - » Cemented total hip arthroplasty

▷ 2-way randomization

    » Reduction and internal fixation

    » Cemented bipolar hemiarthroplasty

▶ Outcome measurements at 4, 12, and 24 months

    ▷ Hip-rating questionnaire (assessed 4 domains: global, pain, walking, and function; initially designed to assess functional outcome of total hip arthroplasty)

    ▷ EQ-5D health status measure

    ▷ Mortality

    ▷ Complications

    ▷ Direct health service costs

▶ 207 patients were enrolled in the 3-way randomization arm.

▶ 91 patients were enrolled in the 2-way randomization arm.

▶ Treatment

    ▷ 118 reduction and fixation

    ▷ 111 bipolar hemiarthroplasty

    ▷ 69 total hip arthroplasty

▶ Average age: 75 years (all patients over age 60).

▶ Not all participants received the operation to which they had been randomly allocated; however, all analyses were based on the allocation groups (the intention-to-treat principle) to avoid biased selection of groups for comparison.

▶ Secondary observational analyses based on the actual operation performed showed a slight widening of the differences observed in the intention-to-treat analyses.

Results

▶ No difference in mortality between the 3 treatment groups.

▶ Secondary surgery

    ▷ 39% in reduction and fixation group

    ▷ 9% in total hip arthroplasty group

    ▷ 5% in bipolar hemiarthroplasty group

▶ Hip rating questionnaire and EQ-5D Scores

    ▷ Worse in the reduction and fixation group at 4 and 12 months

    ▷ Total hip arthroplasty group had significantly better functional outcome scores at 24 months compared to the other 2 groups

▶ Direct costs

▷ Although fixation was initially the least costly procedure, this short-term advantage was eroded by significantly higher costs for subsequent hip-related hospital admissions

Conclusions

▶ Arthroplasty is more clinically effective and cost effective than reduction and fixation in healthy older patients with a displaced intracapsular fracture of the hip.

▶ The long-term results of total hip replacement may be better than those of bipolar hemiarthroplasty.

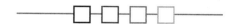

> **FEATURED ARTICLE**
>
> **Authors:** Aharonoff GB, Koval KJ, Skovron ML, Zuckerman JD.
>
> **Title:** Hip fractures in the elderly: predictors of one year mortality.
>
> **Journal Information:** *J Orthop Trauma.* 1997;11(3):162–165.
>
> This is one of the top 20 cited papers published in the *Journal of Orthopaedic Trauma*, 1987 to 2007.

Study Design: Prospective Consecutive Cohort Study

▶ 612 elderly patients with a nonpathologic hip fracture (femoral neck or intertrochanteric)

▷ ≥65 years old

▷ Ambulatory prior to fracture

▷ Lived in their own home (not nursing home residents)

▷ Cognitively intact (moderate to severe dementia were excluded)

Results

▸ 4% (24 patients) died during hospitalization.

▸ 13% (78 patients) died within 1 year of fracture.

▸ Factors predictive of mortality (based on multivariate analysis)

  ▷ Patient age > 85 years

  ▷ Preinjury dependency in basic activities of daily living

  ▷ History of malignancy other than skin cancer

  ▷ American Society of Anesthesiologists rating of operative risk 3 or 4

  ▷ Development of 1 or more in-hospital postop complications

  ▷ All factors other than the development of an in-hospital complication were independent of treatment

Conclusions

▸ Patient age, preinjury dependency in basic activities of daily living, history of malignancy, and American Society of Anesthesiologists rating of operative risk are all independent of treatment.

▸ Efforts at reducing 1-year mortality after hip fracture should be directed at the prevention of postop complications.

▸ This study also provides prognostic information that can be shared with patients and their families.

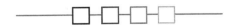

REVIEW ARTICLES

Macaulay W, Pagnotto MR, Iorio R, Mont MA, Saleh KJ. Displaced femoral neck fractures in the elderly: hemiarthroplasty versus total hip arthroplasty. *J Am Acad Orthop Surg.* 2006;14(5):287–293.

Miyamoto RG, Kaplan KM, Levine BR, Egol KA, Zuckerman JD. Surgical management of hip fractures: an evidence-based review of the literature. I: femoral neck fractures. *J Am Acad Orthop Surg.* 2008;16(10):596–607.

Probe R, Ward R. Internal fixation of femoral neck fractures. *J Am Acad Orthop Surg.* 2006;14(9):565–571.

Swiontkowski MF. Current concepts review: intracapsular fractures of the hip. *J Bone Joint Surg Am.* 1994;76-A(1):129–138.

Hip Dislocations

chapter 15

CLASSIC ARTICLE

Authors: Thompson VP, Epstein HC.

Title: Traumatic dislocation of the hip; a survey of two hundred and four cases covering a period of twenty-one years.

Journal Information: *J Bone Joint Surg Am.* 1951;33(3):746–778.

Study Design: Retrospective Review

- 204 traumatic hip dislocations treated from July 1928 to July 1949
  - ▷ 186 (91%) posterior dislocations
  - ▷ 18 (9%) anterior dislocations
- 88 cases were excluded from analysis because of inadequate follow-up, although all patients with fair or poor results with < 1 year follow-up were included.
- 116 were suitable for analysis
  - ▷ 68 cases were examined clinically by 1 or both of the authors
  - ▷ 36 cases were examined by other orthopedic surgeons
  - ▷ 10 cases were examined by other physicians or by personal communication
  - ▷ 2 were not examined clinically
  - ▷ 106 cases had end-result radiographs, while 10 did not
- Average follow-up: 3 years and 9 months (3 months to 19 years).

Hak DJ.
Rapid Reference Review in Orthopedic Trauma: Pivotal Papers Revealed (pp 165-172).
© 2013 SLACK Incorporated.

- ▶ Outcome measurements
  - ▷ Radiographic evaluation
  - ▷ Clinical assessment (excellent, good, fair, poor)
    - » Pain
    - » Hip ROM
    - » Presence or absence of limp
    - » Radiographic results
- ▶ Fracture classification
  - ▷ Type I: no or minor associated fracture
  - ▷ Type II: large single fracture of posterior acetabular rim
  - ▷ Type III: comminuted fracture of posterior acetabular rim, with or without major fragment
  - ▷ Type IV: fracture of acetabular rim and floor
  - ▷ Type V: associated femoral head fracture
- ▶ Acetabular fractures treated nonoperatively with traction.

Results

- ▶ This paper details extensive analysis of numerous different factors on outcome with 18 different tables of variable.
- ▶ Overall results and complications
  - ▷ Anterior dislocation (5 cases)
    - » 5 excellent
    - » No cases of avascular necrosis (AVN), traumatic arthritis, or myositis ossifications
  - ▷ Posterior dislocation type I (30 cases)
    - » 10 excellent
    - » 10 good
    - » 5 fair
    - » 5 poor
    - » 3 developed AVN
    - » 2 developed traumatic arthritis
    - » 1 developed myositis ossificans
  - ▷ Posterior dislocation type II (22 cases)
    - » 7 good
    - » 6 fair
    - » 9 poor
    - » 6 developed AVN

- » 6 developed traumatic arthritis
- » 1 developed myositis ossificans
▷ Posterior dislocation type III (28 cases)
  - » 4 good
  - » 8 fair
  - » 16 poor
  - » 7 developed AVN
  - » 14 developed traumatic arthritis
▷ Posterior dislocation type IV (20 cases)
  - » 1 good
  - » 4 fair
  - » 15 poor
  - » 8 developed AVN
  - » 11 developed traumatic arthritis
▷ Posterior dislocation type V (11 cases)
  - » 1 good
  - » 5 fair
  - » 5 poor
  - » 3 developed AVN
  - » 4 developed traumatic arthritis

Conclusions

▸ AVN and traumatic arthritis were main complications causing unsatisfactory results.

▸ The authors emphasized the importance of prompt recognition of the dislocation and prompt reduction.

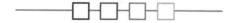

FEATURED ARTICLE

Authors: Schmidt GL, Sciulli R, Altman GT.

Title: Knee injury in patients experiencing a high energy traumatic ipsilateral hip dislocation.

Journal Information: *J Bone Joint Surg Am.* 2005;87(6):1200–1204.

Study Design: Prospective Cohort Study

‣ 28 patients who had a traumatic hip dislocation over a 1-year period.

‣ Investigators evaluated their ipsilateral knee using the following:

  ▷ Standardized history

  ▷ Physical examination

  ▷ Knee MRI

‣ Average age: 39 years (18 to 70 years), 18 males, 10 females.

‣ Mechanism of injury

  ▷ 26 motor vehicle accident

  ▷ 1 crush injury

  ▷ 1 pedestrian accident

‣ 24 (86%) posterior dislocations.

‣ 3 anterior dislocations.

‣ 1 intrapelvic (protrusion) dislocation.

‣ 22 (79%) had an associated acetabular fracture.

Results

‣ 21 (75%) patients reported ipsilateral knee pain.

‣ 11 (39%) were unable to undergo a complete physical examination.

‣ Evidence of major knee ligament injury was present on physical exam in only 2 cases (7%).

‣ 10 (36%) knees had evidence of an effusion on physical exam.

‣ 25 (89%) knees had visible evidence of soft-tissue injury on inspection (abrasion, ecchymosis, contusion, or laceration).

‣ 25 (93%) had positive MRI findings

  ▷ 10 (37%) knee effusions

  ▷ 9 (33%) bone bruises identified

  ▷ 8 (30%) meniscal tears identified

  ▷ 7 (25%) cruciate ligaments (5 posterior cruciate ligaments, 2 anterior cruciate ligaments) injuries identified

  ▷ 6 (21%) collateral ligament injuries identified

  ▷ 4 (14%) periarticular fractures identified

  ▷ 2 (7%) extensor mechanism disruptions identified

Conclusions

‣ There is a high rate of associated ipsilateral knee injuries in patients with a traumatic hip dislocation.

▸ Bone bruises may provide a plausible explanation for persistent knee pain following a traumatic hip dislocation.

▸ The authors recommend the liberal use of MRI to detect knee injuries that may not be discoverable on the basis of a history and physical examination alone.

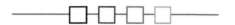

FEATURED ARTICLE

Authors: Dreinhöfer KE, Schwarzkopf SR, Haas NP, Tscherne H.

Title: Isolated traumatic dislocation of the hip. Long-term results in 50 patients.

Journal Information: *J Bone Joint Surg Br.* 1994;76(1):6–12.

Study Design: Retrospective Review

▸ 50 simple hip dislocations (no associated fractures) treated over 15 years.

▸ 38 posterior dislocations.

▸ 12 anterior dislocations.

▸ Average age: 29 years (5 to 62 years), 34 males, 16 females.

▸ All treated by closed reduction under general anesthesia.

▸ 37 patients primarily treated at the authors' hospital

▹ Average time from accident to reduction: 85 minutes (10 to 180 minutes)

▸ 12 patients were primarily treated at other hospitals.

▸ 1 patient was referred with a dislocated hip 8 months after injury.

▸ Associated injuries

▹ 43/50 patients had associated injuries

▹ 14 had multiple severe associated injuries

▸ 7 patients were lost to follow-up, and the 1 late dislocation was excluded from analysis.

▶ Average follow-up of 42 patients: 8 years (2 to 17 years).

▶ Outcome measurements

▷ Radiographs

▷ Objective evaluation according to the Thompson and Epstein (1951) criteria (excellent, good, fair, poor)

Results

▶ Radiographic findings

▷ 2 partial AVN

▷ 7 mild osteoarthritis

▷ 2 moderate degeneration

▷ 4 heterotopic ossification

▶ 29 of 33 MRI examinations were normal.

▶ Thompson and Epstein rating

▷ Anterior dislocations

≫ 75% excellent or good

≫ 25% fair or poor

▷ Posterior dislocations

≫ 47% excellent or good

≫ 53% fair or poor

▶ Patients with no associated injuries

▷ 6/7 had excellent or good result

▶ Patients had severe multiple injuries

▷ 3/8 had excellent or good result

Conclusions

▶ Reduction within 6 hours of injury does not uniformly result in an excellent outcome; rather, it results in a number of long-term complications.

▶ Posterior dislocations are worse than anterior dislocations.

▶ Overall severity of multiple injuries also impacts the long-term prognosis.

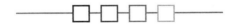

FEATURED ARTICLE

Authors: Sahin V, Karakaş ES, Aksu S, Atlihan D, Turk CY, Halici M.

Title: Traumatic dislocation and fracture-dislocation of the hip: a long-term follow-up study.

Journal Information: *J Trauma*. 2003;54(3):520-529.

Study Design: Retrospective Review

▶ 62 traumatic hip dislocations treated over a 15-year period

  ▷ 57 posterior dislocations

  ▷ 5 anterior dislocations

▶ Average age: 34.5 years (14 to 72 years), 47 males, 15 females.

▶ Mechanism of injury

  ▷ 38 (61%) automobile accidents

  ▷ 5 (8%) motorcycle accidents

  ▷ 9 (15%) pedestrian accidents

  ▷ 8 (13%) work-related injuries

  ▷ 2 (3%) sports injuries

▶ Average follow-up: 9.6 years (3.6 to 18.4 years).

▶ Merle d'Aubigné functional classification (very good, good, medium, fair, and poor).

▶ 71% (4462) had associated injuries.

▶ 50 cases were treated with closed reduction.

▶ 12 cases were treated with open reduction.

▶ 35 hips (56.5%) were reduced within 12 hours of dislocation.

▶ Full weightbearing was resumed an average of 8 weeks (2 to 10 weeks) after injury.

Results

▶ 44 patients (71%) had very good or good to medium results.

▶ 10 patients (16.1%) developed late post-traumatic hip osteoarthritis.

▶ 5 patients (9.6%) developed osteonecrosis of the femoral head.

▶ Significantly better outcomes were seen in patients whose reduction occurred within 12 hours of injury ($P < .05$).

- ▶ Results based on time to reduction
  - ▷ Reduction time ≤ 12 hours
    - » 19 very good
    - » 11 good to medium
    - » 4 fair
    - » 1 poor
    - » 3 developed osteoarthritis
    - » 1 developed AVN
  - ▷ Reduction time > 12 hours
    - » 5 very good
    - » 10 good to medium
    - » 5 fair
    - » 7 poor
    - » 7 developed osteoarthritis
    - » 4 developed AVN

Conclusions

- ▶ Good results can be obtained with early, stable, and accurate reductions by either closed or open methods.
- ▶ The authors recommended that concentric reduction should be confirmed by pelvic radiographs and, if necessary, CT scan.

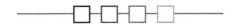

REVIEW ARTICLES

Brooks RA, Ribbans WJ. Diagnosis and imaging studies of traumatic hip dislocations in the adult. *Clin Orthop Relat Res.* 2000;377:15–23.

Clegg TE, Roberts CS, Greene JW, Prather BA. Hip dislocations— epidemiology, treatment, and outcomes. *Injury.* 2010;41(4): 329–334.

Foulk DM, Mullis BH. Hip dislocation: evaluation and management. *J Am Acad Orthop Surg.* 2010;18(4):199–209.

Tornetta P, Mostafavi HR. Hip dislocation: current treatment regimens. *J Am Acad Orthop Surg.* 1997;5(1):27–36.

Acetabular Fractures

chapter **16**

CLASSIC ARTICLE

Authors: Judet R, Judet J, Letornel E.

Title: Fractures of the acetabulum: classification and surgical approach for open reduction—preliminary report.

Journal Information: *J Bone Joint Surg Am.* 1964;46:1615–1646.

Study Design: Retrospective Review

▶ 173 patients sustaining an acetabular fracture
  ▷ 129 treated by ORIF
  ▷ 108 operated on within 3 weeks
  ▷ 21 operated on in a delayed manner
▶ Describes mechanism of injury, radiographic findings, and pathologic findings and outlines a recommended plan of treatment.
▶ Posterior wall fracture was most common pattern (45 cases).
▶ Describes radiographic landmarks seen on AP and Judet (45 degrees oblique) x-rays
  ▷ Iliopectineal line
  ▷ Ilioischial line
  ▷ Tear drop
  ▷ Acetabular roof or dome
  ▷ Anterior lip of acetabulum
  ▷ Posterior lip of acetabulum

Hak DJ.
Rapid Reference Review in Orthopedic Trauma:
Pivotal Papers Revealed (pp 173-183).
© 2013 SLACK Incorporated.

- Describes influence of hip position on acetabular fracture pattern.
- Describes surgical approaches.

Results

- No specific information provided on duration of follow-up; however, they reported
  ▷ 2 cases of AVN
  ▷ 2 cases of severe degenerative arthritis
  ▷ 1 hip ankylosis secondary to infection
  ▷ 5 poor reductions that they anticipate developing degenerative arthritis
  ▷ 3 postop deaths (2 due to pulmonary embolism and 1 due to multiple injuries)

Commentary

- Letournel is widely known for popularizing the surgical treatment of acetabular fractures. This paper, coauthored with his mentor Professor Robert Judet, provides an introduction to the early surgical treatment of acetabular fractures.

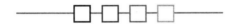

FEATURED ARTICLE
Authors: Giannoudis PV, Grotz MR, Papakostidis C, Dinopoulos H.
Title: Operative treatment of displaced fractures of the acetabulum. A meta-analysis.
Journal Information: *J Bone Joint Surg Br.* 2005;87(1):2–9.

Study Design: Meta-Analysis

- 3670 reported cases of acetabular fracture ORIF to evaluate the following:
  ▷ Classification
  ▷ Incidence of complications
  ▷ Functional outcome of patients
- Average follow-up: 56 months.

Results

▶ Osteoarthritis was the most common long-term complication
  ▷ Overall incidence: 26.6% (reported in 11 studies with 1211 patients)
  ▷ Severe osteoarthritis incidence: 19.1% (111 patients reported in 7 studies with 580 patients)
▶ Heterotopic ossification
  ▷ Overall incidence: 25.6% (reported in 23 studies with 2394 fractures)
  ▷ More severe Brooker III or IV heterotopic ossification incidence: 5.7% (81 cases reported in 13 studies with 1424 patients)
▶ Femoral head avascular necrosis (AVN)
  ▷ Overall incidence of 5.6% (113 patients reported in 18 studies)
▶ Nerve injuries
  ▷ 16.4% incidence of nerve injury at time of admission
  ▷ 8% incidence of iatrogenic postop nerve palsy (194 cases reported in 20 studies with 2426 fractures)
    ≫ >60% involved sciatic nerve (peroneal division)
    ≫ 67 cases involved lateral femoral cutaneous nerve
▶ Secondary operations were only reported in 8% of cases.
▶ 75% to 80% of cases gained excellent or good result at an average of 5 years after injury.
▶ Factors influencing the functional outcome included the following:
  ▷ Type of fracture and/or dislocation
  ▷ Femoral head damage
  ▷ Associated injuries
  ▷ Comorbidity
  ▷ Timing of the operation
  ▷ Surgical approach
  ▷ Reduction quality
  ▷ Local complications

Conclusions

▶ The treatment of these injuries is challenging.
▶ Tertiary referrals need to be undertaken as early as possible because the timing of surgery is of the utmost importance.

▶ It is important to obtain the most accurate fracture reduction possible, with a minimal surgical approach, as both are related to improved outcome.

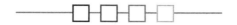

FEATURED ARTICLE

Author: Matta JM.

Title: Fractures of the acetabulum: accuracy of reduction and clinical results in patients managed operatively within three weeks after the injury.

Journal Information: *J Bone Joint Surg Am.* 1996;78(11):1632–1645.

Study Design: Retrospective Review

▶ 262 displaced acetabular fractures (in 259 patients) treated by ORIF within 3 weeks of injury by a single surgeon

  ▷ Patients treated over a period of 11.5 years

  ▷ During this same time, 124 cases of acetabular fracture ORIF were lost to follow-up and were not included in the review

  ▷ During this same period, 57 fractures were treated nonoperatively

▶ 7 fractures followed definitively needed further treatment due to a poor result (less than 2 years from time of ORIF).

▶ Average follow-up of remaining 255 fractures: 6 years (2 to 14 years).

▶ Average age: 37 years (11 to 90 years), 184 males, 75 females.

▶ Fracture classification

  ▷ 21% (54 cases) simple fracture types

    » 1% (3 cases) anterior wall fractures

    » 5% (12 cases) anterior column fractures

    » 8% (22 cases) posterior wall fractures

    » 3% (8 cases) posterior column fractures

    » 3% (9 cases) transverse fractures

▷ 79% (208 cases) associated fracture types

» 35% (92 cases) both column acetabular fractures (the most common pattern)

» 4% (10 cases) posterior column posterior wall fractures

» 23% (61 cases) transverse posterior wall fractures

» 12% (31 cases) T-shaped fractures

» 6% (15 cases) anterior column posterior hemitransverse fractures

▶ Operative approach

▷ 258 operated on through a single approach

» 43% (112 cases) Kocher-Langenbeck approach

» 33% (87 cases) ilioinguinal approach

» 23% (59 cases) extended iliofemoral approach

▷ 4 treated using 2 approaches (Kocher-Langenbeck and ilioinguinal approach)

▶ Outcome measurements

▷ Modified Merle d'Aubigné Score (clinical hip outcome score)

▷ Clinical score based on sum of scores for pain, gait, and hip ROM

▷ Excellent: 18 points

▷ Very good: 16 points

▷ Good: 15 or 16 points

▷ Fair: 13 or 14 points

▷ Poor: < 13 points

▶ Radiographs also measured at time of final follow-up

▷ Excellent: normal-appearing hip joint

▷ Good: mild changes with minimal sclerosis and joint narrowing (≤ 1 mm)

▷ Fair: intermediate changes with moderate sclerosis and joint narrowing (< 50%)

▷ Poor: advanced changes

Results

▶ Reduction accuracy

▷ 71% (185 cases) graded anatomic (0- to 1-mm displacement)

▷ 20% (52 cases) graded imperfect (2- to 3-mm displacement)

▷ 7% (18 cases) graded poor (> 3-mm displacement)

▷ 3% (7 cases) graded secondary congruence (acetabulum anatomic but displaced with respect to innominate bone)

▷ Rate of anatomical reduction decreased with increases in the following:

» Fracture complexity (χ^2 = 44.86; P < .001)

> 96% of simple patterns graded anatomic

> 64% of associated patterns graded anatomic

» Patient age (χ^2 = 37.65; P = .006)

> 78% of patients < 40 years old graded anatomic

> 57% of patients ≥ 40 years old graded anatomic

» Time from injury to ORIF (approached but did not reach statistical significance)

> 74% of cases operated on in first week after injury graded anatomic

> 71% of cases operated on in second week after injury graded anatomic

> 57% of cases operated on in third week after injury graded anatomic

▶ Radiographic grade at final follow-up

▷ 54% (141 hips) excellent (normal-appearing hip joint)

▷ 23% (59 hips) good (mild changes with minimal sclerosis and joint narrowing ≤ 1 mm)

▷ 11% (29 hips) fair (intermediate changes with moderate sclerosis and joint narrowing < 50%)

▷ 13% (33 hips) poor (advanced changes)

▶ Overall clinical result (Merle d'Aubigné Score)

▷ 40% (104 cases) excellent

▷ 36% (95 cases) good

▷ 8% (21 cases) fair

▷ 16% (42) poor

▶ Overall clinical results were closely related to radiographic result.

▶ Overall clinical result was adversely affected by the following:

▷ Femoral head injuries

▷ Older patient age

▷ Operative complications

▶ Overall clinical results positively impacted by the following:

▷ Anatomic reduction

▷ Postop congruity between the femoral head and the acetabular roof

- Complications
  - ▷ 3% (8 cases) femoral head AVN
  - ▷ 5% (13 cases) progressive wear of femoral head
- Subsequent operations
  - ▷ 17 (6%) total hip replacement
  - ▷ 12 (5%) hip arthrodesis
  - ▷ 12 (5%) excision of ectopic bone

Conclusions

- The hip joint can be preserved and post-traumatic osteoarthrosis can be avoided if an anatomical reduction is achieved following complex acetabular fracture.
- The surgeon's goal should be to increase the rate of anatomical reduction and to decrease the rate of operative complications.

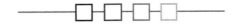

FEATURED ARTICLE
Authors: Moed BR, McMichael JC. **Title:** Outcomes of posterior wall fractures of the acetabulum. **Journal Information:** *J Bone Joint Surg Am.* 2007;89(6): 1170–1176.

Study Design: Retrospective Review

- 46 patients with a minimum 2-year follow-up following posterior wall fracture ORIF.
- Average follow-up: 5 years (2 to 14 years).
- Average age: 36 years (17 to 65 years), 37 males, 9 females.

▶ Outcome measurements
  ▷ Musculoskeletal Function Assessment (MFA)
    » Validated self-reported patient health status questionnaire
    » 10 individual indices and total score
    » MFA scores compared with normative values and with previously reported values for similar patients with hip injuries
  ▷ Modified Merle d'Aubigné Score (clinical hip outcome score)
    » Clinical score based on sum of scores for pain, gait, and hip ROM
    » Excellent: 18 points
    » Very good: 16 points
    » Good: 15 or 16 points
    » Fair: 13 or 14 points
    » Poor: < 13 points

Results

▶ Average Merle d'Aubigné Score: 17 (14 to 18; standard deviation = 1)
  ▷ Overall good-to-excellent clinical results
▶ Average total MFA score: 23.17
  ▷ Significantly worse than the normative average of 9.26 ($P < .001$)
  ▷ All MFA indices except hand/fine motor were significantly worse than expected norms
  ▷ Average MFA total score was statistically similar to that previously reported for patients with hip injuries
  ▷ Emotional category of MFA score was found to be an important determinant of the total score
▶ Negative correlation between the Merle d'Aubigné score and the MFA score ($P < .001$).
▶ Merle d'Aubigné Score data were asymmetric, displaying a ceiling effect (preponderance of scores at the scales' upper end limiting the ability to demonstrate differences between patients with better clinical outcomes).

Conclusions

▶ Total MFA scores following posterior wall fracture ORIF were significantly worse than normative reference values.
▶ Complete recovery after posterior wall fracture ORIF is uncommon, with residual functional deficits involving wide-ranging aspects of everyday living.

- These deficits are not reflected in assessment of hip specific function.
- While the modified Merle d'Aubigné Score may be useful for evaluating isolated hip function following posterior wall ORIF, its shortcomings limit its ability for evaluating patients' functional outcome.

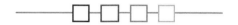

FEATURED ARTICLE
Authors: Moed BR, Carr SE, Gruson KI, Watson JT, Craig JG.
Title: Computed tomographic assessment of fractures of the posterior wall of the acetabulum after operative treatment.
Journal Information: *J Bone Joint Surg Am.* 2003;85-A(3): 512–522.

Study Design: Retrospective Cohort Study

- 67 patients following posterior wall acetabular fracture ORIF with a minimum 2-year follow-up.
- Average age: 40 years (16 to 74 years), 53 males, 14 females.
- 57 patients presented with a hip dislocation
  ▷ 3 hips were irreducible with closed manipulation
- 6 patients were followed to the point of requiring reconstruction surgery due to a poor outcome (at < 2 years).
- Average follow-up of 61 remaining patients: 4 years (2 to 11 years).
- Compared functional results with reduction accuracy.
- Functional outcome measurement
  ▷ Modified Merle d'Aubigné Score (clinical hip outcome score)
    » Clinical score based on sum of scores for pain, gait, and hip ROM
    » Excellent: 18 points
    » Very good: 16 points
    » Good: 15 or 16 points
    » Fair: 13 or 14 points
    » Poor: < 13 points

- Measured reduction accuracy on postop images
  - AP and 2 Judet degrees oblique pelvic radiographs
  - 2-dimensional CT scan
- Radiographs also measured at time of final follow-up
  - Excellent: normal-appearing hip joint
  - Good: mild changes with minimal sclerosis and joint narrowing (≤ 1 mm)
  - Fair: intermediate changes with moderate sclerosis and joint narrowing (< 50%)
  - Poor: advanced changes

Results

- Clinical outcome
  - 46% (31 patients) excellent
  - 30% (20 patients) very good
  - 12% (8 patients) good
  - 12% (8 patients) poor
- Final radiographic results
  - 79% (53 hips) excellent
  - 6% (4 hips) good
  - 5% (3 hips) fair
  - 10% (7 hips) poor
- Strong association between clinical outcome and final radiographic grade.
- Accuracy of fracture reduction as determined with use of plain radiography
  - 65 hips anatomic
  - 2 hips imperfect
- Accuracy of reduction as determined by CT scan
  - 11 hips with incongruency (offset) of > 2 mm
  - 52 hips with fracture gaps ≥ 2 mm
- Fracture gaps ≥ 10 mm in any dimension or a total gap area ≥ 35 mm were associated with a poor result.
- Main risk factors for a poor result were a residual fracture gap width ≥ 10 mm and osteonecrosis of the femoral head.

Conclusions

▶ The degree of residual fracture displacement is detected more accurately on postop CT scans than on plain radiographs.

▶ Accuracy of surgical reduction as assessed on postop CT scan is highly predictive of the clinical outcome.

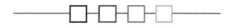

REVIEW ARTICLES

Baumgaertner MR. Fractures of the posterior wall of the acetabulum. *J Am Acad Orthop Surg.* 1999;7(1):54–65.

Letournel E. Acetabulum fractures: classification and management. *Clin Orthop Relat Res.* 1980;151:81–106.

Letournel E. The treatment of acetabular fractures through the ilioinguinal approach. *Clin Orthop Relat Res.* 1993;292:62–76.

Mears DC. Surgical treatment of acetabular fractures in elderly patients with osteoporotic bone. *J Am Acad Orthop Surg.* 1999;7(2):128–141.

Tornetta P III. Displaced acetabular fractures: indications for operative and nonoperative management. *J Am Acad Orthop Surg.* 2001;9(1):18–28.

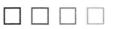

Pelvic Fractures

chapter 17

CLASSIC ARTICLE

Authors: Dalal SA, Burgess AR, Siegel JH, et al.

Title: Pelvic fracture in multiple trauma: classification by mechanism is key to pattern of organ injury, resuscitative requirements, and outcome.

Journal Information: *J Trauma.* 1989;29(7):981–1000.

Study Design: Retrospective Review

▶ 343 multiple-trauma patients with major pelvic ring injuries.

▶ Subdivided patients into 4 major groups based on mechanism of injury

  ▷ Anteroposterior compression (APC)

    ≫ Divided into grades 1 to 3 of increasing severity

  ▷ Lateral compression (LC)

    ≫ Divided into grades 1 to 3 of increasing severity

  ▷ Vertical shear (VS)

  ▷ Combined mechanical injury (CMI) often referred to as *combined mechanism*

Hak DJ.
Rapid Reference Review in Orthopedic Trauma:
Pivotal Papers Revealed (pp 185-195).
© 2013 SLACK Incorporated.

- The pattern of organ injury, complications, and other factors were all evaluated as a function of mortality
  - ▷ Brain, lung, liver, spleen, bowel, and bladder injuries
  - ▷ Pelvic vascular injury
  - ▷ Retroperitoneal hematoma
  - ▷ Circulatory shock
  - ▷ Sepsis
  - ▷ Acute respiratory distress syndrome (ARDS)
  - ▷ Abnormal physiology
  - ▷ 24-hour total fluid volume administration
- Injury mechanism
  - ▷ Motor vehicle accident: 57.4%
  - ▷ Motorcycle accident: 9.3%
  - ▷ Fall: 9.3%
  - ▷ Pedestrian injury: 17.8%
  - ▷ Crush injury: 3.7%

Results

- LC fracture pattern
  - ▷ As grade increased from LC-1 to LC-3, the incidence of pelvic vascular injury, retroperitoneal hematoma, shock, and 24-hour volume needs increased
  - ▷ High incidence of brain, lung, and upper abdominal visceral injuries as causes of death in LC-1 and LC-2
  - ▷ The incidence of brain, lung, and upper abdominal visceral injuries as causes of death actually was lower in LC-3
    - » This discrepancy is explained because most LC-3 injuries were due to severe crush, often being isolated to the pelvis, sparing injury to other organs
- APC fracture pattern
  - ▷ As grade increased from APC-1 to APC-3, the rate of injury to spleen, liver, bowel, pelvic vascular injury with retroperitoneal hematoma, shock, sepsis, and ARDS increased
  - ▷ As grade increased from APC-1 to APC-3, there were large increases in volume needs
  - ▷ High incidence of brain and lung injuries in all APC grades
  - ▷ Mortality rate increased with increasing APC grade
  - ▷ APC-3 had the greatest 24-hour fluid requirements

▶ VS fracture pattern

   ▷ Organ injury pattern similar to severe APC patterns

   ▷ Mortality rate similar to severe APC patterns

▶ Combined mechanism fracture pattern

   ▷ Organ injury pattern similar to lower grades APC and LC patterns

▶ Major differences in the causes of death in LC versus APC injuries

   ▷ Cause of death in LC patterns primarily due to brain injury compounded by shock

   ▷ Cause of death in APC patterns primarily due to shock, sepsis, and ARDS related to the massive torso forces delivered in APC, with large volume losses from visceral organs and pelvis of greater influence in APC

   ▷ Brain injury was not a significant cause of death in APC patterns

Conclusions

▶ The mechanical force type and severity of the pelvic fracture are the keys to the expected organ injury pattern, resuscitation needs, and mortality.

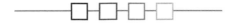

FEATURED ARTICLE

Authors: Burgess AR, Eastridge BJ, Young JW, et al.

Title: Pelvic ring disruptions: effective classification system and treatment protocols.

Journal Information: *J Trauma.* 1990;30(7):848–856.

Study Design: Retrospective Review

▶ 210 consecutive high-energy pelvic ring injuries treated at Maryland Shock Trauma Center from January 1985 to September 1988.

▶ 162/210 patients had complete charts/records available for review.

▶ Treated by a standard protocol based on the patient's pelvic injury classification and hemodynamic status.

- Injury classification based on the vector of force involved and the quantification of disruption from that force
  ▷ APC
  ▷ LC
  ▷ VS
  ▷ CMI often referred to as combined mechanism
- 15% (25/162) were admitted in shock with a blood pressure < 90 mm Hg.
- Average Injury Severity Score: 26 (4 to 75).
- Pelvic fracture treatments (alone or in combination)
  ▷ Acute external fixation (45/162, 28.0%)
  ▷ ORIF (22/162, 14%)
  ▷ Acute arterial embolization (11/162, 7.0%)
  ▷ Bed rest (68/162, 42.0%)
- Overall average blood replacement: 5.9 units
  ▷ APC average blood replacement: 14.8 units
  ▷ VS average blood replacement: 9.2 units
  ▷ Combined mechanical average blood replacement: 8.5 units
  ▷ LC average blood replacement: 3.6 units
- Overall mortality: 8.6%
  ▷ APC: 20%
  ▷ Combined mechanical: 18%
  ▷ LC: 7%
  ▷ VS: 0%
  ▷ The cause of death was associated with the pelvic fracture in less than 50%

Conclusions

- The predictive value of our classification system (incorporating appreciation of the causative forces and resulting injury patterns) and their classification-based treatment protocols reduced the morbidity and mortality related to pelvic ring injuries.

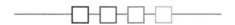

FEATURED ARTICLE

Authors: Routt ML Jr, Simonian PT, Mills WJ.

Title: Iliosacral screw fixation: early complications of the percutaneous technique.

Journal Information: *J Orthop Trauma.* 1997;11(8):584–589.

This is one of the top 20 cited papers published in the *Journal of Orthopaedic Trauma*, 1987 to 2007.

Study Design: Prospective Cohort Study

▸ 177 consecutive patients with displaced unstable pelvic ring disruptions treated with percutaneous iliosacral screws.

▸ Average age: 32 years (11 to 78 years), 102 males, 75 females.

▸ Anterior pelvic ring reduction and fixation was performed by internal and external fixation techniques.

▸ Accurate closed or open reductions of the posterior pelvic ring disruption were achieved using a variety of surgical techniques

  ▷ Closed manipulative reduction of the posterior pelvic ring was attempted in all patients

  ▷ If closed manipulation was unsuccessful (more than 1 cm residual displacement in any field of fluoroscopic imaging), open reduction was performed

▸ Both postop plain radiographs and postop CT scans were evaluated.

Results

▸ Minimal blood loss.

▸ Complications

  ▷ Due to inadequate imaging

    » Fluoroscopic imaging was inadequate due to obesity or abdominal contrast in 18 patients

  ▷ Due to surgeon error

    » 5 screws were misplaced due to surgeon error

    » 1 misplaced screw caused a transient L-5 neuropraxia

  ▷ Due to fixation failure

    » 7 patients

▸ 2 sacral nonunions that required débridement, bone grafting, and repeat fixation.

Conclusions

▸ Iliosacral screw fixation of the posterior pelvis is difficult, and the surgeon must understand the variability of sacral anatomy.

▸ Quality triplanar fluoroscopic imaging of the accurately reduced posterior pelvic ring should allow for safe iliosacral screw insertions.

▸ Anticipated noncompliant patients or those with craniocerebral trauma may need supplementary posterior pelvic fixation.

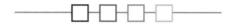

FEATURED ARTICLE

Authors: Matta JM, Tornetta P III.

Title: Internal fixation of unstable pelvic ring injuries.

Journal Information: *Clin Orthop Relat Res.* 1996;329:129–140.

Study Design: Retrospective Review

▸ 107 unstable pelvic fractures treated operatively.

▸ Minimum 6 months follow-up.

▸ 31 patients had only anterior fixation.

▸ 69 patients had unilateral posterior fixation.

▸ 7 patients had bilateral posterior fixation.

▸ Reductions were graded by the maximal displacement measured on the 3 standard pelvic views (AP, inlet, and outlet)
  ▹ Excellent: ≤ 4 mm residual displacement
  ▹ Good: 5 to 10 mm residual displacement
  ▹ Fair: 10 to 20 mm residual displacement
  ▹ Poor > 20 mm residual displacement

Results

▶ Reduction quality

▷ 72 excellent

▷ 30 good

▷ 4 fair

▷ 1 poor

▶ ORIFs within 21 days of injury were associated with a higher percentage of excellent reductions than in reductions performed after 21 days (70% versus 55%), but these differences were not statistically significant.

▶ Operative complications

▷ 1 femoral vein laceration

▷ 1 bladder laceration

▷ 4 broken drill bits

▷ 3 wound hematomas

▷ 1 transient L-5 neuropraxia

▶ 3 deep infections.

Conclusions

▶ The authors recommended use of a single 6-hole curved 3.5-mm reconstruction plate for anterior fixation of unstable pelvic ring injuries.

▶ Rami fractures are usually stable after posterior fixation

▷ Most rami fractures are due to LC injuries, leaving the ilioinguinal ligament intact, which helps maintain reduction of the rami fracture following posterior fixation

▶ Rami fixation should only be considered in severely displaced fractures.

Commentary

▶ This article provides several excellent diagrams that illustrate the use of various clamps to achieve reduction of displaced pelvic ring injuries.

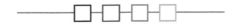

FEATURED ARTICLE

Authors: Sagi HC, Papp S.

Title: Comparative radiographic and clinical outcome of two-hole and multi-hole symphyseal plating.

Journal Information: *J Orthop Trauma.* 2008;22(6):373–378.

Study Design: Retrospective Study

- Chart and radiographic review of 92 patients who underwent anterior pelvic ring ORIF using different anterior plates (surgeon randomized)
  - 51 patients treated with a 2-hole 4.5-mm plate
  - 41 patients treated with a multihole plate (minimum of 2 4.5-mm screws on either side of the symphysis)
- There was a similar pattern of injury distribution and posterior ring fixation between the 2 groups.
- Average age: 44 years (19 to 77 years).
- The endpoint for follow-up was one of the following:
  - A clinically healed injury (defined as discharge from further follow-up)
  - Malunion
  - Fixation failure
  - Reoperation on the anterior ring
  - Actual duration of follow-up not specified
- Malunion was defined as >5-mm displacement of the hemipelvis and pubic symphysis in a nonanatomic position, either rotational or translational.

Results

- Significantly greater failure rate in the cases fixed with a 2-hole plate (*P* = .018)
  - 33% (17/51) failure rate in the 2-hole plate group
  - 12% (5/41) failure rate in the multihole plate group
- Significantly greater malunion rate in the cases fixed with a 2-hole plate (*P* = .001)
  - 57% (29/51) malunion rate in the 2-hole plate group
  - 15% (6/41) malunion rate in the multihole plate group

- No significant difference in reoperation rates between the 2 groups (*P* = .666)
  - ▷ 16% (8/51) in the 2-hole plate group
  - ▷ 12% (5/41) in the multihole plate group

Conclusions

- The authors recommend the use of a multihole plate for fixation of the anterior pelvic ring because it is associated with a lower failure rate and a lower rate of pelvic malunion.

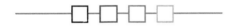

FEATURED ARTICLE

Authors: Putnis SE, Pearce R, Wali UJ, Bircher MD, Rickman MS.

Title: Open reduction and internal fixation of a traumatic diastasis of the pubic symphysis: one-year radiological and functional outcomes.

Journal Information: *J Bone Joint Surg Br.* 2011;93(1):78–84.

Study Design: Retrospective Review

- 49 out of 52 consecutive patients who underwent ORIF of traumatic pubic symphysis diastasis.
- Average age: 42 years (18 to 70 years), 41 males, 8 females.
- Outcome measurements at 1 year
  - ▷ SF-12
  - ▷ 6 questions specific to pelvic injury that reported on the type, location, and frequency of pelvic pain and how it affected their physical function during the prior 4 weeks
- Radiographs taken at 3, 6, and 12 months.

Results

- No postop wound infections.
- 31% (15/49) had radiographic signs of anterior pelvic plate and screw movement
  ▷ 11 cases were seen at 3 months postop
  ▷ 3 additional cases were seen at 6 months postop
  ▷ 1 additional case was seen at 12 months postop
- 12% (6/49) had loss of reduction and recurrent symphysis diastasis
  ▷ 4 of these cases underwent revision surgery due to anterior pain
  ▷ 2 had good functional outcomes despite the recurrent diastasis and required no additional surgery
- Functional outcome measurements were available for 41 of the 49 patients
  ▷ 14/15 patients who had hardware loosening completed outcome measurements
  ▷ 27/34 patients without hardware loosening completed outcome measurements
- Mental health SF-12 was similar to the normal population (study group 49.5 versus 50 for normal).
- Physical health SF-12 was lower, but not statistically different than the normal population (study group 42.5 versus 50 for normal).
- Pain levels at 1 year
  ▷ 37% (15/41) pain free
  ▷ 29% (12/41) mild or very mild pain
  ▷ 27% (11/41) moderate pain
  ▷ 7% (3/41) severe pain
- There was no significant difference in the SF-12 scores and levels of pain in the 11 patients with radiographic evidence of hardware movement who did not require revision surgery compared to the rest of the group
  ▷ SF-12 physical score (P = .12)
    » 50.2 in hardware movement group
    » 42.5 in the rest of the group
  ▷ SF-12 mental health score (P = .46)
    » 52.2 in hardware movement group
    » 49.5 in the rest of the group

▷ No difference in level of pain between the groups (*P* = .32)

» Levels of pain in 11 patients with radiographic evidence of hardware movement who did not require revision surgery

⟩ 45% (5/11) no pain

⟩ 36% (4/11) mild or very mild pain

⟩ 18% (2/11) moderate pain

Conclusions

▸ The radiographic appearance of anterior fixation movement is common.

▸ Radiographic appearance of anterior fixation movement by itself is not an indication for revision surgery.

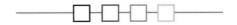

REVIEW ARTICLES

Hak DJ, Smith WR, Suzuki T. Management of hemorrhage in life-threatening pelvic fracture. *J Am Acad Orthop Surg.* 2009;17(7):447–457.

Mehta S, Auerbach JD, Born CT, Chin KR. Sacral fractures. *J Am Acad Orthop Surg.* 2006;14(12):656–665.

Papathanasopoulos A, Tzioupis C, Giannoudis VP, Roberts C, Giannoudis PV. Biomechanical aspects of pelvic ring reconstruction techniques: evidence today. *Injury.* 2010;41(12): 1220–1227.

Tile M. Acute pelvic fractures: I. Causation and classification. *J Am Acad Orthop Surg.* 1996;4(3):143–151.

Tile M. Acute pelvic fractures: II. Principles of management. *J Am Acad Orthop Surg.* 1996;4(3):152–161.

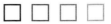

Distal Radius Fractures

chapter **18**

CLASSIC ARTICLE

Authors: Knirk JL, Jupiter JB.

Title: Intra-articular fractures of the distal end of the radius in young adults.

Journal Information: *J Bone Joint Surg Am.* 1986;68(5):647–659.

Study Design: Retrospective Case Series

▸ 43 distal radius fractures in 40 young adults

　▷ Average age: 27.6 years (19 to 39 years)

▸ Fracture treatment

　▷ 21 closed reduction and cast

　▷ 17 closed reduction, Kirschner wire (K-wire) fixation, and cast

　▷ 2 external fixations

　▷ 3 ORIF

▸ Outcome measure

　▷ Gartland and Werley demerit scale system (Sarmiento modification)—includes residual deformity, subjective evaluation, objective evaluation, and radiographic appearance

▸ Average follow-up: 6.7 years.

Results

- 26% excellent (Gartland and Werley Score 0 to 2).
- 35% good (Gartland and Werley Score 3 to 8).
- 33% fair (Gartland and Werley Score 9 to 20).
- 6% poor (Gartland and Werley Score ≥ 21).
- Presence of post-traumatic arthritis correlated strongly with poorer assessment using the Gartland and Werley demerit scale system.
- Post-traumatic arthritis present in 65% of wrists
  - ▷ Arthritis present in 91% of 24 fractures that healed with articular incongruity
  - ▷ Arthritis present in only 11% of the 19 fractures that healed with a congruous joint
- Depressed articular surface (die-punch fragment) was reduced anatomically by closed means in only 49% and was responsible for articular incongruity in 75% of the incongruous joints at late follow-up.
- Prognostic factors that influenced development of post-traumatic arthritis
  - ▷ Failure to obtain and/or maintain articular congruity
  - ▷ Extent of initial disruption
  - ▷ Initial dorsal angulation or radial length
  - ▷ Maintenance of final reduction

Conclusions

- Accurate articular restoration was the most critical factor in achieving a successful result.

Commentary

- This remains a classic article that details the critical importance of reduction for good functional outcome in young patients. While the surgical techniques have advanced since the time of this article (more frequent internal fixation), the observations and conclusions of this article remain valid.

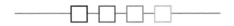

FEATURED ARTICLE

Authors: Grewal R, Perey B, Wilmik M, Stothers K.

Title: A randomized prospective study on the treatment of intraarticular distal radius fractures: open reduction and internal fixation with dorsal plating versus mini open reduction, percutaneous fixation, and external fixation.

Journal Information: *J Hand Surg.* 2005;30(4):764–772.

Study Design: Prospective, Randomized Study

▶ 62 patients with intra-articular distal radius fractures (AO type C) randomized

  ▷ 29 patients randomized to ORIF with dorsal plating ("Pi" plate, Synthes, Paoli, PA)

    » Pi plate designed to overcome prior plate limitations

    » Lower profile to decrease extensor tendon irritation

    » Locking screws to improve fixation in osteoporotic bone

  ▷ 33 patients randomized to mini open reduction with percutaneous K-wire and external fixation

▶ Excluded patients > 70 years, any associated soft-tissue or skeletal injury to the same limb, and pre-existing wrist arthrosis or disability.

▶ Average follow-up: 18 months (6 to 24 months).

▶ 8 patients were lost to follow-up

  ▷ 3 patients in dorsal plate group were lost to follow-up

  ▷ 5 patients in ORIF group were lost to follow-up

▶ Objective, subjective, and radiographic outcomes were assessed at 2 weeks, 4 to 6 weeks, 10 to 12 weeks, 6 months, and 1- and 2-year intervals.

▶ Primary outcome measurement

  ▷ Disabilities of the Arm, Shoulder, and Hand (DASH) Score

▶ Secondary outcome measurements

  ▷ Grip strength

  ▷ ROM

  ▷ Surgical procedure time

  ▷ Complications

  ▷ Radiographic parameters measurements

▸ Groups were equal with respect to age, gender, fracture subtype, and number of Workers' Compensation cases.

Results

▸ No significant difference between the 2 groups in the DASH Score.

▸ Dorsal plate group had a significantly higher complication rate (P = .004)
  ▷ 17 patients in the dorsal plate group experienced 21 complications (72.4% complication rate)
    ≫ 3 reflex sympathetic dystrophy
    ≫ 1 compartment syndrome
    ≫ 5 tendinitis
    ≫ 3 sensory impairments
    ≫ 1 patient required ulnar-shortening osteotomy
    ≫ 8 hardware removals
  ▷ 8 patients in the external fixation group experienced 8 complications (24.2% complication rate)
    ≫ 2 reflex sympathetic dystrophy
    ≫ 1 distal radioulnar joint instability
    ≫ 1 sensory loss
    ≫ 1 stiff hand complaint
    ≫ 2 pin track infections
    ≫ 1 patient required ulnar-shortening osteotomy

▸ Dorsal plate group had significantly longer surgical times (P = .02)
  ▷ Dorsal plate group average surgical time: 105 minutes
  ▷ External fixator group average surgical time: 71 minutes

▸ Dorsal plate group had significantly longer tourniquet times (P < .001)
  ▷ Dorsal plate group average tourniquet time: 82 minutes
  ▷ External fixator group average tourniquet time: 52 minutes

▸ Dorsal plate group had higher pain levels at 1 year (P = .02); however, this equalized after hardware removal.
  ▷ Average DASH pain subcategory score at 1 year
    ≫ Dorsal plate group: 22
    ≫ External fixator group: 10
  ▷ Average DASH pain subcategory score at 2 years not significantly different (P = .47)
    ≫ Dorsal plate group: 11 (8 patients had undergone removal of painful plates)
    ≫ External fixator group: 9

- External fixator group had significantly better grip strength (P = .019)
  - ▷ 97% in external fixator group (compared with the normal side)
  - ▷ 86% in dorsal plate group (compared with the normal side)

Conclusions

- At mid-term analysis of the study, the dorsal plate group showed a significantly higher complication rate, and therefore, further enrollment in the study was terminated.
- Because the dorsal plate group showed statistically significantly higher levels of pain, weaker grip strength, and longer surgical and tourniquet times, the investigators could not recommend the use of dorsal plates for treatment of complex intra-articular distal radius fractures.

Commentary

- While the dorsal plate is no longer commonly used, this paper provides important historical perspective on the evolution of distal radius fracture treatment.

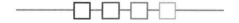

FEATURED ARTICLE

Authors: Kreder HJ, Hanel DP, Agel J, et al.

Title: Indirect reduction and percutaneous fixation versus open reduction and internal fixation for displaced intraarticular fractures of the distal radius: a randomised, controlled trial.

Journal Information: *J Bone Joint Surg Br.* 2005;87(6):829–836.

Study Design: Prospective Randomized Study

- 179 adult patients with displaced intra-articular distal radius fractures
  - ▷ 88 patients randomized to indirect percutaneous reduction and external fixation
  - ▷ 91 patients randomized to ORIF through either volar or dorsal approach with fixation by small or mini-fragment plates
- Follow-up
  - ▷ 166 (93%) completed 6-months follow-up

▷ 140 (78%) completed 1-year follow-up

▷ 118 (66%) completed 2-year follow-up

▸ Primary outcome measurements

  ▷ Upper limb Musculoskeletal Function Assessment (MFA)

  ▷ SF-36

▸ Secondary outcome measurements

  ▷ Jebsen hand function test

  ▷ Pinch strength

  ▷ Grip strength

Results

▸ Significant improvements in all patients in both groups during the first year, including the following:

  ▷ Upper limb MFA Score

  ▷ SF-36 bodily pain subscale score

  ▷ Overall Jebsen score

  ▷ Pinch strength

  ▷ Grip strength

▸ At 6 months, they found better overall function in the indirect percutaneous reduction and external fixation group, scoring an average 6 points better on upper limb MFA.

▸ However, at 12 and 24 months, there was no difference in the upper limb MFA scores.

▸ A repeated-measures analysis was used to consider overall difference between the treatment groups over the entire period of evaluation rather than at an isolated time point

  ▷ Repeated-measures analysis of variance (ANOVA) favored indirect percutaneous reduction and external fixation over ORIF

▸ No statistically significant difference in radiological anatomic reduction.

▸ No statistically significant difference in the ROM.

Conclusions

▸ Patients who underwent indirect reduction and percutaneous fixation had a more rapid return of function and a better functional outcome than those who underwent ORIF provided that the intra-articular step and gap deformity were minimized.

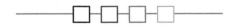

FEATURED ARTICLE

Authors: Kreder HJ, Agel J, Mckee MD, Schemitsch EH, Stephen D, Hanel DP.

Title: A randomized, controlled trial of distal radius fractures with metaphyseal displacement but without joint incongruity: closed reduction and casting versus closed reduction, spanning external fixation, and optional percutaneous K-wires.

Journal Information: *J Orthop Trauma.* 2006;20(2):115–121.

Study Design: Prospective Randomized Multicenter (3 University Teaching Hospitals) Study

▸ 113 patients with distal radius fractures with metaphyseal displacement but without joint incongruity

  ▷ 59 randomized to closed reduction and casting

  ▷ 54 randomized to closed reduction and external fixation with optional K-wire fixation

▸ Outcome measurements

  ▷ Upper extremity MFA

  ▷ Jebsen Taylor scores

  ▷ Pinch strength

  ▷ Grip strength

  ▷ SF-36 to evaluate global function and pain

  ▷ Radiographic evaluation

  ▷ ROM

▸ Follow-up

  ▷ 108 (96%) completed 6-month follow-up

  ▷ 94 (83%) completed 1-year follow-up

  ▷ 85 (75%) completed 2-year follow-up

Results

▸ While there was a trend for better function in the external fixation group at all time points, this did not reach statistical significance.

▸ There was also a trend for better length and palmar tilt restoration with external fixation, but this did not reach statistical significance.

- Upper extremity MFA scores, Jebsen Taylor scores, SF-36 bodily pain scores, and grip strength improved significantly during the first year in all patients.
- At 2 years, the average Jebsen Taylor scores and SF-36 bodily pain scores for patients in both groups were similar to scores for normal age- and gender-matched population controls.

Conclusions

- Investigators showed a trend for better functional, clinical, and radiographic outcomes when those displaced without joint incongruity are treated with external fixation.
- Given the observed difference, they estimated that a sample size of 600 patients in each group would be required to demonstrate statistical significance.

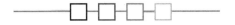

INITIAL REPORT FROM
VOLAR LOCKING PLATE DESIGNER

Author: Orbay JL.

Title: The treatment of unstable distal radius fractures with volar fixation.

Journal Information: *Hand Surg.* 2000;5(2):103–112.

Study Design: Retrospective Review

- 29 patients with 31 unstable distal radius fractures treated by ORIF with a locked volar plate.
- Introduced the use of a volar locking distal radius plate that provides stable fixation and allows early motion while avoiding the complications seen with dorsal plate fixation.
- Describes surgical technique.
- Most had failed closed reduction and casting; 3 had failed external fixation.

- Fracture pattern
  - ▷ 14 intra-articular fractures
  - ▷ 17 extra-articular fractures
- Average age: 54 years (25 to 86 years).
- Preop radiographs
  - ▷ Average dorsal tilt: 30 degrees (0 to 65 degrees)
  - ▷ Average radial inclination: 10 degrees (–10 to 25 degrees)
  - ▷ Average radial shortening: 3 mm (0 to 8 mm)
- Cancellous allograft was used in 3 patients to fill large metaphyseal voids.
- Average follow-up: 66 weeks (53 to 98 weeks).

Results

- Radiographic
  - ▷ Average palmar tilt: 5 degrees (5 degrees dorsal tilt to 8 degrees volar tilt)
  - ▷ Average radial inclination: 21 degrees (18 to 26 degrees)
  - ▷ Average radial shortening: 1 mm (0 to 2 mm)
  - ▷ Average articular incongruity: 0 mm (0 to 1 mm)
- No measurable loss of reduction after plating.
- No plate breakage.
- 10 patients required physical therapy, while the other 19 performed independent rehabilitation.
- Wrist motion
  - ▷ Average wrist extension: 59 degrees (45 to 85 degrees)
  - ▷ Average wrist flexion: 57 degrees (40 to 80 degrees)
  - ▷ Average ulnar deviation: 27 degrees (15 to 40 degrees)
  - ▷ Average radial deviation: 17 degrees (10 to 25 degrees)
  - ▷ Average pronation: 80 degrees (65 to 90 degrees)
  - ▷ Average supination: 78 degrees (70 to 90 degrees)
- Grip strength averages 79% contralateral side (60% to 110%).
- Functional outcome according to Gartland and Werley scale
  - ▷ 19 excellent
  - ▷ 12 good
- Complications
  - ▷ 1 dorsal tendon irritation from an excessively long peg
  - ▷ 3 patients underwent hardware removal

Conclusions

▶ Volar locking plate offers several advantages compared to other treatment methods of unstable distal radius fractures, including the following:

▷ Elimination of most dorsal tendon irritation

▷ Improved pronation and supination due to release of pronator quadratus, which is commonly trapped in the fracture site

▷ Prompt functional recovery and reduced need for therapy

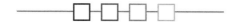

REVIEW ARTICLES

Berglund LM, Messer TM. Complications of volar plate fixation for managing distal radius fractures. *J Am Acad Orthop Surg.* 2009;17(6):369–377.

Henry MH. Distal radius fractures: current concepts. *J Hand Surg.* 2008;33(7):1215–1227.

Jupiter JB. Complex articular fractures of the distal radius: classification and management. *J Am Acad Orthop Surg.* 1997; 5(3):119–129.

Lichtman DM, Bindra RR, Boyer MI, et al. AAOS clinical practice guideline summary: treatment of distal radius fractures. *J Am Acad Orthop Surg.* 2010;18(3):180–189.

Nana AD, Joshi A, Lichtman DM. Plating of the distal radius. *J Am Acad Orthop Surg.* 2005;13(3):159–171.

Orbay JL, Touhami A. Current concepts in volar fixed-angle fixation of unstable distal radius fractures. *Clin Orthop Relat Res.* 2006;445:58–67.

Smith DW, Henry MH. Volar fixed-angle plating of the distal radius. *J Am Acad Orthop Surg.* 2005;13(1):28–36.

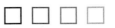

Forearm Fractures

chapter **19**

CLASSIC ARTICLE

Authors: Chapman MW, Gordon JE, Zissimos AG.

Title: Compression-plate fixation of acute fractures of the diaphyses of the radius and ulna.

Journal Information: *J Bone Joint Surg Am*. 1989;71(2):159–169.

Study Design: Retrospective Study

▶ 129 diaphyseal forearm fractures with a minimum 1-year follow-up.

▶ Average age: 33 years (13 to 79 years).

▶ Implants

▷ 117 fractures (91%) treated with a 3.5-mm AO dynamic compression plate (DCP)

▷ 3 fractures treated with 4.5-mm AO narrow DCP

▷ 9 treated with semitubular or third-tubular plate

▶ Both open and comminuted fractures were routinely bone grafted.

▶ Outcome evaluation (after Anderson et al, *J Bone Joint Surg Am.* 1975;57[3]:287–297.)

▷ Excellent defined as union with less than 10 degrees loss of wrist or elbow flexion or extension and less than 25% loss of pronation/ supination

Hak DJ.
Rapid Reference Review in Orthopedic Trauma: Pivotal Papers Revealed (pp 207-212).
© 2013 SLACK Incorporated.

▷ Satisfactory defined as union with less than 20 degrees loss of wrist or elbow flexion or extension and less than 50% loss of pronation/supination

▷ Unsatisfactory defined as union with either more than 20 degrees loss of wrist or elbow flexion or extension or more than 50% loss of pronation/supination

▷ Failure defined as nonunion or unresolved chronic osteomyelitis

Results

▸ 98% union rate.

▸ 92% excellent or satisfactory results.

▸ 2 patients had early loss of fixation, both of the ulna.

▸ 2.3% infection rate.

▸ 34 plates were symptomatic and were removed after fracture union.

▸ Refractures

▷ Zero following removal of 3.5-mm DCP, third-tubular, or semitubular implants

▷ Both bones fractured from which a 4.5-mm narrow DCP was removed

Conclusions

▸ Immediate plate fixation of open forearm fractures possible with a low infection rate

▷ In contrast, in series by Anderson and colleagues (*J Bone Joint Surg Am.* 1975;57[3]:287–297). ORIF of open fractures was delayed

▸ Risk of refracture following removal is low with 3.5-mm implants.

▸ High risk of refracture following removal with use of 4.5-mm implants.

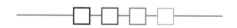

FEATURED ARTICLE
Authors: Anderson LD, Sisk D, Tooms RE, Park WI III.
Title: Compression-plate fixation in acute diaphyseal fractures of the radius and ulna.
Journal Information: *J Bone Joint Surg Am.* 1975;57(3):287–297.

Study Design: Retrospective Review

- ▶ 244 patients with 330 acute diaphyseal fractures of the radius and ulna treated with compression plates between 1960 and 1970
  - ▷ 216 patients had closed injuries
  - ▷ 28 patients had open injuries
  - ▷ 112 patients had both bone fractures
  - ▷ 50 patients had isolated ulnar shaft fractures
  - ▷ 82 patients had isolated radial shaft fractures
- ▶ Follow-up range: 4 months to 9 years.
- ▶ Outcome evaluation
  - ▷ Excellent defined as union with less than 10 degrees loss of wrist or elbow flexion or extension and less than 25% loss of pronation/supination
  - ▷ Satisfactory defined as union with less than 20 degrees loss of wrist or elbow flexion or extension and less than 50% loss of pronation/supination
  - ▷ Unsatisfactory defined as union with either more than 20 degrees loss of wrist or elbow flexion or extension or more than 50% loss of pronation/supination
  - ▷ Failure defined as nonunion or unresolved chronic osteomyelitis

Operative Technique

- ▶ Authors noted that the periosteum is not stripped; instead, the muscle is dissected carefully away from the periosteum, disturbing it as little as possible to minimize bony blood supply damage.
- ▶ The AO group recommends that the screws engage at least 5 cortices in each of the main fragments.
- ▶ Compression achieved using outrigger compression device, as this was prior to the widespread use of the dynamic compression plate.
- ▶ 63 patients (26%) with severely comminuted fractures had iliac crest bone grafting.
- ▶ ORIF was delayed in all open fractures to be certain that infection was not present (average delay: 10.6 days, range: 1 to 3 weeks).

Results

- ▶ 97.9% union rate for radius.
- ▶ 96.3% union rate for ulna.
- ▶ Function was rated excellent or satisfactory in 85% and unsatisfactory in 15%.

Conclusions

▶ AO compression plates provided a successful method for obtaining union and restoring optimum function after acute diaphyseal forearm fractures.

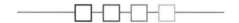

FEATURED ARTICLE
Authors: Hidaka S, Gustilo RB. **Title:** Refracture of bones of the forearm after plate removal. **Journal Information:** *J Bone Joint Surg Am.* 1984;66(8):1241–243.

Study Design: Retrospective Review

▶ 32 forearm plates removed from 23 patients between 1977 and 1982
  ▷ 18 ulnar plates
  ▷ 14 radial plates
  ▷ 22 plates were elective removals
  ▷ 11 plates were removed for pain
▶ Time from application to removal ranged from 8 to 62 months.
▶ Patients were protected by cast immobilization for an average of 6 weeks after plate removal.

Results

▶ 7 refractures (22%)—This rate was significantly higher than the 1% to 1.5% reported in *AO Manual of Internal Fixation*, 2nd edition, 1979
  ▷ 6 patients had a refracture of the radius
  ▷ 1 patient had a refracture of the radius and ulna

▷ Fracture site

» 3 occurred through prior fracture site

» 3 occurred through prior fracture site and extended into an adjacent screw hole

» 1 occurred through a screw hole

▸ Refractures occurred between 2 and 40 weeks after plate removal.

Conclusions

▸ If a plate has to be removed, the authors recommended use of a protective splint, brace, or functional cast for at least a few weeks afterward.

▸ The authors also recommended restriction of athletic activity, heavy lifting, and torsional stresses for 1 year.

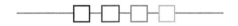

FEATURED ARTICLE

Authors: Leung F, Chow SP.

Title: A prospective, randomized trial comparing the limited contact dynamic compression plate with the point contact fixator for forearm fractures.

Journal Information: *J Bone Joint Surg Am.* 2003;85-A(12): 2343–2348.

Study Design: Prospective Randomized Study

▸ 92 patients with 125 forearm fractures (65 radial shaft fractures, 60 ulnar shaft fractures)

▷ 47 patients randomized to treatment with limited contact dynamic compression plate (LC-DCP)

▷ 45 patients randomized to treatment with point contact fixator (PC-Fix [Depuy Synthes, West Chester, PA]), which was an early version of a locking plate

- Average patient age: 36 years (11 to 90 years).
- Average follow-up: 22 months.

Results

- No significant difference in operative time, time to union, callus formation, pain, or functional outcome.
- No nonunions.
- 4 fractures (3 patients) in the PC-Fix group and 5 fractures (5 patients) in LC-DCP group were a delayed union.
- 1 deep infection occurred in a closed fracture in the PC-Fix group and 1 in an open fracture in the LC-DCP group.
- Plate removal
  - ▷ At the time of the final follow-up, 22 PC-Fix and 29 LC-DCP implants had been removed from 37 patients (average: 15 months between insertion and removal)
  - ▷ One refracture occurred in each group, both at a screw hole site

Conclusions

- Despite the differences in the concept of fracture fixation, these 2 implants appear to be equally effective for the treatment of diaphyseal forearm fracture.

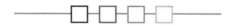

REVIEW ARTICLES
Bhandari M, Schemitsch EH. Fractures of the shaft of the ulna. *J Orthop Trauma.* 2004;18(7):473–475.
Moss JP, Bynum DK. Diaphyseal fractures of the radius and ulna in adults. *Hand Clin.* 2007;23(2):143–151.
Sauder DJ, Athwal GS. Management of isolated ulnar shaft fractures. *Hand Clin.* 2007;23(2):179–184.

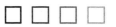

Radial Head Fractures

chapter *20*

CLASSIC ARTICLE

Authors: Broberg MA, Morrey BF.

Title: Results of delayed excision of the radial head after fracture.

Journal Information: *J Bone Joint Surg Am.* 1986;68(5):669–674.

Study Design: Retrospective Review

▶ 21 patients who underwent delayed excision of a previously fractured radial head.

▶ Time from fracture to excision (1 month to more than 20 years).

▶ Fracture classification
  ▷ 4 Mason II
  ▷ 17 Mason III
  ▷ 5 fractures were associated with an elbow dislocation

▶ Average follow-up from excision: 15 years (3 to 32 years).

▶ Evaluation by personal interview, examination, and testing in an upper-extremity biomechanics laboratory
  ▷ Pain
  ▷ Motion
  ▷ Strength
  ▷ Stability
  ▷ Functional Rating Index (used in several subsequent papers)

Hak DJ.
Rapid Reference Review in Orthopedic Trauma:
Pivotal Papers Revealed (pp 213-220).
© 2013 SLACK Incorporated.

- Broberg and Morrey Functional Rating Index
  - ▷ Motion
    - » Flexion (0 to 27 point scale)
    - » Pronation (0 to 6 point scale)
    - » Supination (0 to 7 point scale)
  - ▷ Strength (0 to 20 point scale)
  - ▷ Stability (0 to 5 point scare)
  - ▷ Pain (0 to 35 point scale)
  - ▷ Excellent: 95 to 100 points
  - ▷ Good: 80 to 94 points
  - ▷ Fair: 69 to 79 points
  - ▷ Poor: 0 to 59 points

Results

- Pain improved following radial head excision in 76% of patients
  - ▷ No patients had any increase in pain following excision
- Both flexion and rotation following radial head excision in 81% of patients
  - ▷ Average preop flexion arc: 27 to 118 degrees
  - ▷ Average postop flexion arc: 18 to 135 degrees
  - ▷ 3 patients lost 5 to 20 degrees of extension following excision
  - ▷ Average preop pronation: 39 degrees
  - ▷ Average postop pronation: 62 degrees
  - ▷ Average preop supination: 40 degrees
  - ▷ Average postop supination: 68 degrees
- Functional index score
  - ▷ 77% good or excellent
  - ▷ 23% fair or poor

Conclusions

- Delayed excision after failure of closed management of fractures of the radial head is successful in relieving pain and improving motion.
- The authors suggested that this justified initial closed treatment of radial head fractures, with delayed excision of the radial head to be considered as needed.
- Prior to this, many authors advocated immediate excision, some even recommending excision within 24 hours of injury.

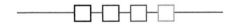

FEATURED ARTICLE

Authors: Ikeda M, Sugiyama K, Kang C, Takagaki T, Oka Y.

Title: Comminuted fractures of the radial head. Comparison of resection and internal fixation.

Journal Information: *J Bone Joint Surg Am.* 2005;87(1):76–84.

Study Design: Retrospective Review

- 28 patients with Mason III radial head fractures
  - 15 had been treated by radial head excision
    - » Average follow-up: 10 years
  - 13 had been treated by ORIF
    - » Average follow-up: 3 years
  - Prior to 1996, their primary treatment for comminuted radial head fractures was radial head excision
  - After 1996, their primary treatment was ORIF whenever possible
- Outcomes assessment
  - Pain
  - Motion
  - Radiographic findings
  - Strength as measured by Cybex testing
  - Broberg and Morrey Functional Rating Index
  - American Shoulder and Elbow Surgeons Elbow Assessment Form

Results

- Pain (25 points representing the best score)
  - Average: 19.3 (12 to 25) in resection group
  - Average: 22.4 (17 to 25) in ORIF group ($P = .0226$)
- Motion
  - ROM in the 2 groups was similar
  - The degree of flexion contracture was significantly higher in the resection group (15.5 versus 7.1 degrees, $P = .0254$)
  - Average motion: 15.5 degrees (flexion contracture) to 131.4 degrees (flexion) in the resection group
  - Average motion: 7.1 degrees (flexion contracture) to 133.8 degrees (flexion) in the ORIF group

- Strength
  - ▷ The radial head resection group had a greater loss of strength in extension, pronation, and supination ($P < .01$)
- Broberg and Morrey functional rating score (higher score is better)
  - ▷ 81.4 in resection group
    - » 9 good, 5 fair, 1 poor
  - ▷ 90.7 in ORIF group ($P = .0034$)
    - » 3 excellent, 9 good, 1 fair
- American Shoulder and Elbow Surgeons Elbow Assessment Score
  - ▷ 87.3 in resection group
  - ▷ 94.6 in ORIF group ($P = .0031$)

Conclusions

- ORIF is the treatment of choice when feasible.
- ORIF group had satisfactory joint motion, with greater strength and better function than patients treated by radial head excision.

Commentary

- One major limitation of this paper is the marked difference in follow-up duration between the 2 groups, although all of the ORIF patients did have a minimum 2-year follow-up.

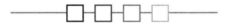

FEATURED ARTICLE

Authors: Ring D, Quintero J, Jupiter JB.

Title: Open reduction and internal fixation of fractures of the radial head.

Journal Information: *J Bone Joint Surg Am.* 2002;84-A(10): 1811–1815.

Study Design: Retrospective Review

▶ 56 patients with intra-articular radial head fractures treated by ORIF at 2 institutions from January 1990 to January 1997.

▶ Average age: 36 years (17 to 62 years), 35 males, 21 females.

▶ Average follow-up: 48 months (all had a 24-month minimum follow-up).

▶ Classification

▷ 30 Mason II (partial articular)

» 15 were comminuted

▷ 26 Mason III (complete articular)

» 14 were comminuted with more than 3 fragments

» 12 had 2 or 3 fragments

▶ 27 cases were associated with a fracture-dislocation or an injury to the medial collateral ligament.

▶ Definition of unsatisfactory results

▷ Early failure of fixation

▷ Nonunion requiring additional surgery for radial head excision

▷ < 100 degrees of forearm rotation

▷ Fair or poor rating based on Broberg and Morrey system

Results

▶ 4/15 comminuted Mason II fractures had unsatisfactory results

▷ All were associated with elbow fracture-dislocation

▷ All had < 100 degrees of forearm motion

▶ All 15 noncomminuted Mason II fractures had satisfactory results.

▶ 13/14 comminuted Mason III fractures had unsatisfactory results.

▶ 1/12 Mason III fractures with 2 or 3 fragments had unsatisfactory results due to a nonunion.

Conclusions

▶ ORIF is best reserved for minimally comminuted fractures with 3 or fewer articular fragments.

▶ Associated fracture-dislocation of the elbow or forearm may also compromise the long-term result of radial head repair, especially with regard to restoration of forearm rotation.

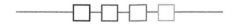

FEATURED ARTICLE

Authors: Moro JK, Werier J, MacDermid JC, Patterson SD, King GJ.

Title: Arthroplasty with a metal radial head for unreconstructible fractures of the radial head.

Journal Information: *J Bone Joint Surg Am.* 2001;83-A(8): 1201–1211.

Study Design: Retrospective Review

▸ 25 unreconstructable fractures of the radial head in 24 consecutive patients treated with a metal radial heal arthroplasty.

▸ Average age: 54 years (27 to 84 years).

▸ Minimum 2-year follow-up, average follow-up: 39 months (26 to 58 months).

▸ Fracture classification

   ▷ 10 Mason II

   ▷ 15 Mason-Johnston IV

▸ 2 were isolated injuries, and 23 were associated with other elbow fracture and/or ligamentous injuries.

▸ Assessment

   ▷ Clinical exam including ROM and strength

   ▷ Radiographic exam

   ▷ SF-36

      ≫ Standardized to the overall US population with an average score of 50

   ▷ Disabilities of the Arm, Shoulder, and Hand Questionnaire (DASH)

   ▷ American Shoulder and Elbow Surgeons Elbow Assessment Form

   ▷ Mayo Elbow Performance Index (MEPI)

   ▷ Patient-Rated Wrist Evaluation

   ▷ Wrist Outcome Score

Results

▸ SF-36 summary scores suggested that overall health-related quality of life was within the normal range (physical component = 47 ± 10; mental component = 49 ± 13).

- Other outcome scales indicated mild disability of the upper extremity
  ▷ DASH = 17 ± 19
  ▷ Patient-Rated Wrist Evaluation Score = 17 ± 21
  ▷ Wrist Outcome Score = 60 ± 10
  ▷ MEPI = 80 ± 16
- MEPI
  ▷ 17 good or excellent
  ▷ 5 fair
  ▷ 3 poor
- Subjective patient satisfaction averaged 9.2 on a scale of 1 to 10.
- ROM
  ▷ Elbow flexion of the injured extremity averaged 140 ± 9 degrees
  ▷ Elbow extension: −8 ± 7 degrees
  ▷ Pronation: 78 ± 9 degrees
  ▷ Supination: 68 ± 10 degrees
- A significant loss of elbow flexion and extension and forearm supination occurred in the affected extremity, which also had significantly less strength of isometric forearm (17%) and supination (18%) as well as significantly less grip strength ($P < .05$).
- Asymptomatic bone lucencies surrounded the stem of the implant in 17 of the 25 elbows.
- Valgus stability was restored, and proximal radial migration did not occur.
- Complication
  ▷ 1 complex regional pain syndrome
  ▷ 1 ulnar neuropathy
  ▷ 1 posterior interosseous nerve palsy
  ▷ 1 episode of elbow stiffness
  ▷ 1 wound infection

Conclusions

- Patients with a comminuted radial head fracture treated with a metal radial head implant will have mild-to-moderate impairment of the physical capability of the elbow and wrist.

▶ At the time of short-term follow-up, arthroplasty with a metal radial head implant was found to be safe and effective for unreconstructable radial head fracture.

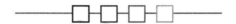

REVIEW ARTICLES

Hotchkiss RN. Displaced fractures of the radial head: internal fixation or excision? *Am Acad Orthop Surg.* 1997;5(1):1–10.

Mathew PK, Athwal GS, King GJ. Terrible triad injury of the elbow: current concepts. *J Am Acad Orthop Surg.* 2009;17(3):137–151.

Tejwani NC, Mehta H. Fractures of the radial head and neck: current concepts in management. *J Am Acad Orthop Surg.* 2007;15(7):380–387.

Olecranon Fractures

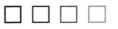

chapter **21**

FEATURED ARTICLE

Authors: Hume MC, Wiss DA.

Title: Olecranon fractures. A clinical and radiographic comparison of tension band wiring and plate fixation.

Journal Information: *Clin Orthop Relat Res.* 1992;285:229–235.

Study Design: Prospective, Randomized Study

▸ 41 patients with displaced olecranon fractures

  ▷ 19 patients randomized to tension band wiring

  ▷ 22 patients randomized to plate fixation (third-tubular small fragment nonlocking plate)

▸ Average age: 31 years (18 to 67 years), 30 males, 11 females.

▸ Outcome assessments

  ▷ Clinical assessment

    » Good: No more than slight or occasional pain, loss of elbow motion < 15 degrees

    » Fair: Occasional to moderate pain, loss of elbow motion of 15 to 30 degrees

    » Poor: Constant pain, loss of elbow motion > 30 degrees, operative failures requiring revision

Hak DJ.
*Rapid Reference Review in Orthopedic Trauma:
Pivotal Papers Revealed (pp 221-226).*
© 2013 SLACK Incorporated.

  ▷ Radiographic assessment

    » Good: No articular step-off or gap, no loss of reduction

    » Fair: Articular step-off or gap < 2 mm, no loss of reduction

    » Poor: Articular step-off or gap > 2 mm or loss of reduction

▸ Average follow-up: 28.5 weeks (16 to 86 weeks).

Results

▸ Longer operative time in the plate fixation group

  ▷ Average operative time for tension band wiring: 94.5 minutes (75 to 120 minutes)

  ▷ Average operative time for plate fixation: 120 minutes (85 to 150 minutes)

▸ No significant difference in elbow motion between the 2 groups.

▸ Symptomatic hardware

  ▷ 42% (8/19) in tension band wiring group, although Kirschner wire (K-wire) migration seen in only 1 case

  ▷ 5% (1/22) in plate fixation group

▸ Postop loss of reduction leading to a significant articular step-off or gap

  ▷ 53% (10/19) of tension band wiring cases

  ▷ 5% (1/22) of plate fixation cases

▸ Clinical results

  ▷ Good

    » 47% (9/19) with tension band wiring

    » 86% (19/22) with plate fixation

  ▷ Fair

    » 32% (6/19) with tension band wiring

    » 5% (1/22) with plate fixation

  ▷ Poor

    » 21% (4/19) with tension band wiring

    » 9% (2/22) with plate fixation

▸ Radiographic results

  ▷ Good

    » 37% (7/19) with tension band wiring

    » 64% (14/22) with plate fixation

▷ Fair

  » 10% (2/19) with tension band wiring

  » 27% (6/22) with plate fixation

▷ Poor

  » 53% (10/19) with tension band wiring

  » 9% (2/22) with plate fixation

Conclusions

▶ The authors recommended that plate fixation should be strongly considered when planning ORIF of displaced olecranon fractures.

▶ In this study, plate fixation resulted in more anatomic reductions and better maintenance of reduction.

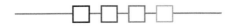

FEATURED ARTICLE

Authors: Macko D, Szabo RM.

Title: Complications of tension-band wiring of olecranon fractures.

Journal Information: *J Bone Joint Surg Am.* 1985;67(9): 1396–1401.

Study Design: Retrospective Review

▶ 20 patients with olecranon fractures treated by tension band wiring out of 30 total patients treated over a 6-year period.

▶ Average age: 35.5 years (15 to 76 years).

▶ Average follow-up: 13.5 months (3 to 50 months).

▶ Outcome graded according to ROM and presence of pain

  ▷ Excellent: < 5 degrees loss of flexion/extension, full pronation and supination, and no pain

  ▷ Good: 5 to 20 degrees loss of flexion/extension, full pronation and supination, and no pain

▷ Fair: 40 degrees of useful flexion-extension, ≤ 10 degrees loss of pronation/supination, and no pain

▷ Poor: Pain or < 40 degrees of useful flexion-extension

Results

▸ Symptomatic prominent hardware was present in 16/20 patients.

▸ 4 patients had skin breakdown due to the prominent hardware.

▸ 1 patient had associated soft-tissue infection.

▸ Migration of wires occurred in only 3 patients

▷ Average migration: 4 mm (2 to 5 mm)

▸ The majority of prominent hardware was due to inadequate seating at time of surgery.

▸ 2 fractures lost reduction.

▸ Hardware removal was performed in 12 patients.

▸ Outcome grading

▷ 9 excellent

▷ 7 good

▷ 3 fair

▷ 1 poor

Conclusions

▸ Most complications that are related to this method of fixation may be avoided by careful attention to surgical technique.

▸ The authors noted the importance of placing the tension band wire deep to the triceps tendon and on the periosteum of the olecranon and bending the proximal ends of the K-wires 180 degrees and inserting them flush with the cortex of the proximal fragment.

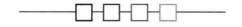

FEATURED ARTICLE

Authors: Chalidis BE, Sachinis NC, Samoladas EP, Dimitriou CG, Pournaras JD.

Title: Is tension band wiring technique the "gold standard" for the treatment of olecranon fractures? A long term functional outcome study.

Journal Information: *J Orthop Surg Res.* 2008;3:9.

Study Design: Retrospective Review

▶ 62 isolated olecranon fractures treated with tension band wiring.

▶ Average age: 48.6 years (18 to 85 years), 33 males, 29 females.

▶ Higher prevalence of fractures in males until the fifth decade.

▶ Higher prevalence of fractures in females from the sixth decade onward.

▶ 61% (38/62) were due to simple falls, while 39% (24/62) were due to high-energy injuries.

▶ Average follow-up: 8 years (6 to 13 years).

▶ Clinical assessment for ROM.

▶ Radiographic assessment.

▶ Functional outcome assessment
  ▷ Mayo Elbow Performance Score (MEPS)
  ▷ VAS subjective pain score
  ▷ VAS patient satisfaction score

Results

▶ Hardware removal performed in 82% (51/62) of cases.

▶ 67% (34/51) who had undergone removal still complained of mild pain during daily activities.

▶ Supination was more affected than pronation ($P = .027$).

▸ MEPS

▷ 53 (85%) patients had a good or excellent result

▷ 6 (10%) fair

▷ 3 (5%) poor

▸ Average satisfaction rating: 9.3 (6 to 10)

▷ 31 patients (50%) completely satisfied

▸ Degenerative radiographic changes noted in 30 elbows (48%), but these changes showed no correlation with the MEPS ($P = .073$).

Conclusions

▸ The authors concluded that tension band wiring fixation remains the "gold standard" for the treatment of displaced and minimally comminuted olecranon fractures.

▸ They noted that in the long term, low levels of pain may be present regardless of whether hardware has been removed or whether degenerative changes have developed.

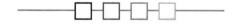

REVIEW ARTICLES

Hak DJ, Golladay GJ. Olecranon fractures: treatment options. *J Am Acad Orthop Surg*. 2000;8(4):266–275.

Newman SD, Mauffrey C, Krikler S. Olecranon fractures. *Injury*. 2009;40(6):575–581.

Veillette CJ, Steinmann SP. Olecranon fractures. *Orthop Clin North Am*. 2008;39(2):229–236.

Elbow Dislocations

chapter 22

FEATURED ARTICLE

Authors: Josefsson PO, Gentz CF, Johnell O, Wenderberg B.

Title: Surgical versus non-surgical treatment of ligamentous injuries following dislocation of the elbow joint. A prospective randomized study.

Journal Information: *J Bone Joint Surg Am.* 1987;69(4):605–608.

Study Design: Prospective Randomized Study

▸ 30 consecutive patients with a simple elbow dislocation (no concomitant fracture).

▸ All patients examined under general anesthesia
  ▷ 15 randomized to surgical treatment
  ▷ 15 randomized to nonsurgical treatment

▸ Elbow findings at time of initial exam under anesthesia
  ▷ 30 had medial instability
  ▷ 16 had both medial and lateral instability

▸ All of the surgically treated elbows showed complete rupture or avulsion of both the medial and lateral collateral ligaments
  ▷ In about half of these patients, the muscle origins were found to be torn from the humeral epicondyles

▸ Follow-up available on 28/30 patients.

Hak DJ.
*Rapid Reference Review in Orthopedic Trauma:
Pivotal Papers Revealed (pp 227-232).*
© 2013 SLACK Incorporated.

- Average follow-up
  - ▷ 31 months (14 to 59 months) in surgical treatment group
  - ▷ 24 months (12 to 48 months) in nonsurgical treatment group

Results

- Both treatment groups showed good results.
- Differences between the groups were not statistically significant.

Conclusions

- There is no evidence that the results of surgical ligament repair were any better than those with nonsurgical treatment.

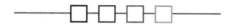

FEATURED ARTICLE

Authors: Rafai M, Largab A, Cohen D, Trafeh M.

Title: Luxation posterieure pure du coude chez l'adulte: immobilisation ou mobilisation precoce. Etude prospective randomisee sur 50 cas. [Pure posterior dislocation of the elbow in adults: Plaster immobilization or early mobilization. Randomized prospective study of 50 cases.]

Journal Information: *Chir Main.* 1999;18(4):272–278.

Study Design: Prospective Randomized Study

- 50 pure posterior elbow dislocations
  - ▷ 26 randomized to reduction under general anesthesia and plaster immobilization for 3 weeks, followed by rehabilitation
  - ▷ 24 randomized to reduction under general anesthesia, followed by early mobilization

Results

- ▶ Better recovery of elbow function in patients treated by early mobilization
  - ▷ 96% good results with recovery of normal extension in patients treated with early mobilization
  - ▷ 81% good results in patients treated with 3 weeks of plaster immobilization
- ▶ Significantly lower rate of stiffness in the early mobilization group
  - ▷ 4% of patients in the early mobilization group had stiffness
  - ▷ 19% of patients treated with 3 weeks of plaster immobilization had stiffness
  - ▷ Incomplete recovery of extension at 12 months
    - » 1/24 in early mobilization group
    - » 5/26 in 3-week plaster mobilization group
  - ▷ Incomplete recovery of flexion at 12 months
    - » 1/24 in early mobilization group
    - » 5/26 in 3-week plaster mobilization group
  - ▷ Incomplete recovery of pronation/supination at 12 months
    - » 1/24 in early mobilization group
    - » 5/26 in 3-week plaster mobilization group
- ▶ No significant difference in residual pain between the 2 treatment groups
  - » 1/24 in early mobilization group
  - » 1/26 in 3-week plaster mobilization group
- ▶ No recurrences of dislocation, instability, or heterotopic ossifications were observed in either groups

Conclusions

- ▶ Early mobilization following a simple elbow dislocation is superior to 3 weeks of plaster immobilization.
- ▶ Early mobilization allows recovery of better elbow function without increasing the risk of elbow instability or recurrent dislocation.

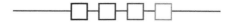

FEATURED ARTICLE

Authors: Maripuri SN, Debnath UK, Rao P, Mohanty K.

Title: Simple elbow dislocation among adults: a comparative study of two different methods of treatment.

Journal Information: *Injury.* 2007;38(11):1254–1258.

Study Design: Retrospective Cohort Review

▸ 42 simple elbow dislocations (no associated fracture).
▸ Patient treatment
  ▷ 20 patients treated by splint immobilization for an average of 2 weeks followed by physical therapy
  ▷ 22 patients treated with a sling followed by early mobilization
▸ Minimum follow-up: 2 years (2 to 5 years).
▸ Outcome measurements
  ▷ Mayo Elbow Performance Index (MEPI)
  ▷ Quick Disabilities of the Arm, Shoulder, and Hand (DASH) questionnaire

Results

▸ MEPI Score
  ▷ Splint immobilization group
    » 10 excellent
    » 2 good
    » 5 fair
    » 3 poor
  ▷ Sling and early mobilization group
    » 19 excellent
    » 1 good
    » 2 fair
▸ Average MEPI Score significantly better in sling and early mobilization group ($P < .05$)
  ▷ 83.8 in splint immobilization group
  ▷ 96.5 in sling and early mobilization group

- Average Quick DASH Score significantly better in sling and early mobilization group (*P* < .05)
  - ▷ 12.8 in splint immobilization group
  - ▷ 2.7 in sling and early mobilization group
- Average time to return to work significantly different (*P* < .001)
  - ▷ 6.6 weeks in splint immobilization group
  - ▷ 3.2 weeks in the sling and early mobilization group
- Duration of physical therapy was longer in the splint immobilization group.
- No redislocations or late instability in the early mobilization group.

Conclusions

- Early active mobilization is a safe and cost-effective method for treatment of simple elbow dislocations.
- Early active mobilization results in significantly better final functional outcome than initial short-term splint immobilization.

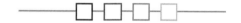

FEATURED ARTICLE

Authors: Schippinger G, Seibert FJ, Steinböck J, Kucharczyk M.

Title: Management of simple elbow dislocations. Does the period of immobilization affect the eventual results?

Journal Information: *Langenbecks Arch Surg.* 1999;384(3): 294–297.

Study Design: Retrospective Cohort Study

- 45 patients with simple elbow dislocations.
- Average follow-up: 61.5 months (18 to 84 months).
- Outcome measurements
  - ▷ ROM
  - ▷ Radiographic evaluation
  - ▷ Morrey Elbow Score used to evaluate pain, limitation of motion, instability, and daily activities

- For analysis, patients were divided into 3 groups based on the duration of immobilization
  ▷ < 2 weeks
  ▷ 2 to 3 weeks
  ▷ > 3 weeks

Results

- Overall results were good or excellent with regard to pain and function.
- Loss of terminal extension was the most common finding
  ▷ 9% had a flexion contracture > 10 to 30 degrees
  ▷ 36% had a flexion contracture < 10 degrees
- Periarticular ossification was seen in 28 patients (62%) but did not lead to loss of motion.
- There was no statistical difference between the 3 groups of immobilization, but better results were seen in patients immobilized for less than 3 weeks compared to those immobilized for more than 3 weeks.

Conclusions

- Splint immobilization for 2 weeks enhances patient comfort and does not adversely affect the eventual outcome.
- Splint immobilization for more than 3 weeks may result in worse function.

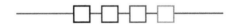

REVIEW ARTICLES

Cohen MS, Hastings H II. Acute elbow dislocation: evaluation and management. *J Am Acad Orthop Surg.* 1998;6(1):15–23.

Hobgood ER, Khan SO, Field LD. Acute dislocations of the adult elbow. *Hand Clin.* 2008;24(1):1–7.

Mathew PK, Athwal GS, King GJW. Terrible triad injury of the elbow: current concepts. *J Am Acad Orthop Surg.* 2009;17(3):137–151.

Tashjian RZ, Katarincic JA. Complex elbow instability. *J Am Acad Orthop Surg.* 2006;14(5):278-286.

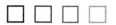

Supracondylar Humerus Fractures

chapter *23*

CLASSIC ARTICLE

Authors: Jupiter JB, Neff U, Holzach P, Allgöwer M.

Title: Intercondylar fractures of the humerus: an operative approach.

Journal Information: *J Bone Joint Surg Am.* 1985;67(2):226–239.

Study Design: Retrospective Review

▶ 34 intra-articular supracondylar humerus fractures treated by ORIF between 1968 and 1978 in Basel, Switzerland.

▶ Average age: 57 years (17 to 79 years), 18 males, 16 females.

▶ Fracture classification

  ▷ 13 type C1

  ▷ 2 type C2

  ▷ 19 type C3

▶ 14 (41%) fractures were open injuries (9 grade I, 4 grade II, 1 grade III).

▶ Average follow-up: 5.8 years (2 to 12 years).

▶ Evaluation

  ▷ Written questionnaire of subjective symptoms

  ▷ Physical examination

    » Excellent: ROM from 15 degrees flexion contracture to 130 degrees flexion

    » Good: 30 degrees flexion contracture to 120 degrees flexion

Hak DJ.
Rapid Reference Review in Orthopedic Trauma:
Pivotal Papers Revealed (pp 233-240).
© 2013 SLACK Incorporated.

» Fair: 40 degrees flexion contracture to 90 to 120 degrees flexion

» Poor: 40 degrees flexion contracture to < 90 degrees flexion

▷ Combined subjective symptoms rating with ROM to provide overall functional rating

▷ Radiographs

▸ Operative technique

▷ Olecranon osteotomy performed in 26/34 patients

▷ Reduction of articular surface

▷ Reduction of reconstructed articular surface to shaft

▷ Fixation with 1 or 2 third-tubular or semitubular small fragment plates

Results

▸ 13 Excellent

▷ Normal or nearly normal motion

▷ No pain

▷ No disability

▸ 14 Good

▷ Slight limitation in motion

▷ Occasional pain

▷ Minimal disability

▸ 4 Fair

▷ Moderate limitation in motion

▷ Pain with activity

▷ Moderate disability

▸ 3 Poor

▷ Marked limitation in motion

▷ Variable pain

▷ Severe disability

▷ All 3 poor results were in multiple trauma patients, and 2 had type C3 fractures.

▸ Complications

▷ 5 postop neuritis

▷ 3 nonunions

▷ 1 refracture

▷ 1 heterotopic ossification

▷ 1 deep infection

Conclusions

▶ The operative approach is technically demanding and is best attempted by a surgeon experienced in the approach and well-versed in ORIF.

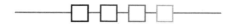

FEATURED ARTICLE

Authors: McKee MD, Veillette CJ, Hall JA, et al.

Title: A multicenter, prospective, randomized, controlled trial of open reduction—internal fixation versus total elbow arthroplasty for displaced intra-articular distal humeral fractures in elderly patients.

Journal Information: *J Shoulder Elbow Surg.* 2009;18(1):3–12.

Study Design: Prospective, Randomized (by Sealed Envelope), Controlled Trial

▶ 42 elderly patients (age >65) with displaced intra-articular distal humeral fractures

  ▷ 21 patients randomized to ORIF

    » 5 patients randomized to ORIF were converted to total elbow arthroplasty (TEA) intraoperatively because of comminution and inability to obtain stable internal fixation

  ▷ 21 patients randomized to semiconstrained TEA

▶ 2 patients died prior to follow-up and were excluded.

▶ 15 patients in final ORIF group

  ▷ Average age: 77 years, 3 males, 12 females

▶ 25 patients in final elbow arthroplasty group

  ▷ Average age: 78 years, 2 males, 23 females

▶ Outcomes assessment at 6 weeks and 3, 6, 12, and 24 months

  ▷ Mayo Elbow Performance Score (MEPS)

  ▷ Disabilities of the Arm, Shoulder, and Hand (DASH)

Results

▶ Operative time averaged 32 minutes less in the TEA group (P = .001).

▶ Elbow arthroplasty patients had significantly better MEPS at 3 months (83 versus 65, P = .01), 6 months (86 versus 68, P = .003), 12 months (88 versus 72, P = .007), and 2 years (86 versus 73, P = .015) compared with the ORIF group.

▶ Elbow arthroplasty patients had significantly better DASH Scores at 6 weeks (43 versus 77, P = .02) and 6 months (31 versus 50, P = .01) but not at 12 months (32 versus 47, P = .1) or 2 years (34 versus 38, P = .6).

▶ No significant difference in average flexion-extension arc (P = .19)

  ▷ TEA group average flexion-extension arc: 107 degrees (42 to 145 degrees)

  ▷ ORIF group average flexion-extension arc: 95 degrees (30 to 140 degrees)

▶ No significant difference in reoperation rate (P = .20)

  ▷ 3/25 (12%) reoperations in TEA group

  ▷ 4/15 (27%) reoperations in ORIF group

Conclusions

▶ TEA is a preferred alternative for ORIF in elderly patients with complex distal humeral fractures that are not amenable to stable fixation.

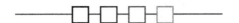

FEATURED ARTICLE

Authors: Ring D, Jupiter JB, Gulotta L.

Title: Articular fractures of the distal part of the humerus.

Journal Information: *J Bone Joint Surg Am.* 2003;85-A(2): 232–238.

Study Design: Retrospective Review

▸ 21 patients with an articular fracture of the distal part of the humerus.

▸ Reviewed at an average of 40 months after injury.

▸ Identified 5 components of the injury to evaluate the patterns of fracture

   ▷ Capitellum and the lateral aspect of the trochlea

   ▷ Lateral epicondyle

   ▷ Posterior aspect of the lateral column

   ▷ Posterior aspect of the trochlea

   ▷ Medial epicondyle

Results

▸ All fractures healed, and no patient had residual ulnohumeral instability or weakness.

▸ 10 patients required a second operation

   ▷ 6 for release of an elbow contracture

   ▷ 2 for treatment of ulnar neuropathy

   ▷ 1 removal of symptomatic hardware

   ▷ 1 for early loss of fixation

▸ Average arc of ulnohumeral motion: 96 degrees (55 to 140 degrees).

▸ Mayo Elbow Performance Index (MEPI) Scores

   ▷ 4 excellent

   ▷ 12 good

   ▷ 5 fair

Conclusions

▸ Apparent fractures of the capitellum are often more complex fractures of the articular surface of the distal part of the humerus.

▸ Treatment of these injuries with operative reduction and fixation with buried implants can result in satisfactory restoration of elbow function.

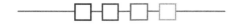

FEATURED ARTICLE

Authors: Doornberg JN, van Duijn PJ, Linzel D, et al.

Title: Surgical treatment of intra-articular fractures of the distal part of the humerus. Functional outcome after twelve to thirty years.

Journal Information: *J Bone Joint Surg Am.* 2007;89(7): 1524–1532.

▸ This study investigated the long-term clinical and radiographic results following ORIF of intra-articular distal humerus fractures.

▸ 30 patients.

▸ Average follow-up: 19 years (12 to 30 years).

Results

▸ Excluding 1 elbow requiring arthrodesis (counted as a poor result), the average final flexion arc was 106 degrees, and the average pronation-supination arc was 165 degrees.

▸ Average American Shoulder and Elbow Surgeons (ASES) Score was 96 points.

▸ Average satisfaction score was 8.8 points on a 0- to 10-point VAS.

▸ Average DASH Score was 7 points.

▸ Average MEPI Score was 91 points.

▸ Including the patient with the arthrodesis, the final categorical ratings were as follows:

  ▷ 19 excellent

  ▷ 7 good

  ▷ 1 fair

  ▷ 3 poor

▸ The radiographic appearance of arthrosis did not appear to correlate with pain or predict disability or function.

▸ Subsequent procedures were performed in 12 patients (40%).

Conclusions

▸ The long-term results of intra-articular distal humerus fracture ORIF were similar to those reported for the short term.

▶ Functional ratings and perceived disability were predicated more on pain than on functional impairment and did not correlate with radiographic signs of arthrosis.

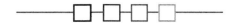

FEATURED ARTICLE

Authors: McKee MD, Jupiter JB, Bamberger HB.

Title: Coronal shear fractures of the distal end of the humerus.

Journal Information: *J Bone Joint Surg Am.* 1996;78(1):49–54.

Study Design: Retrospective Review

▶ 6 patients with shear fracture of the distal articular surface of the humerus, with anterior and proximal displacement of the capitellum and a portion of the trochlea.

▶ Fracture classification

▷ Type 1 (the Hahn-Steinthal fracture) involves most of the capitellum, with little or no extension into the lateral aspect of the trochlea

▷ Type 2 (the Kocher-Lorenz fracture) involves only the anterior cartilage of the capitellum, with a thin layer of subchondral bone

▷ Type 3, described by Broberg and Morrey, is a comminuted fracture of the capitellum

▶ Average age: 38 years (10 to 63 years), 1 male, 5 females.

▶ Identified characteristic radiographic abnormality on lateral radiograph that they termed the *double-arc* sign

▷ Represents the subchondral bone of the displaced capitellum and the lateral trochlear ridge

▶ All patients treated by ORIF with early motion.

▶ Average follow-up: 22 months (18 to 26 months).

▶ Outcomes assessment

▷ Broberg and Morrey Functional Rating Index (strength, motion, stability, and pain)

▷ Radiographic findings

Results

- ► All fractures united without evidence of osteonecrosis.
- ► ROM
  - ▷ Average elbow flexion: 141 degrees (130 to 150 degrees)
  - ▷ Average elbow flexion contracture: 15 degrees (0 to 40 degrees)
  - ▷ Average pronation: 83 degrees (50 to 90 degrees)
  - ▷ Average supination: 84 degrees (55 to 90 degrees)
- ► Broberg and Morrey elbow rating score
  - ▷ All good or excellent functional results

Conclusions

- ► Despite the limited soft-tissue attachments on these displaced articular fracture fragments, osteonecrosis is not likely to occur.
- ► Although these fractures are difficult to recognize and to reduce accurately, rigid fixation and early motion reliably restore elbow function.

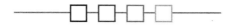

REVIEW ARTICLES

Anglen J. Surgical techniques: distal humerus fractures. *J Am Acad Orthop Surg.* 2005;13(5):291–297.

Galano GJ, Ahmad CS, Levine WN. Current treatment strategies for bicolumnar distal humerus fractures. *J Am Acad Orthop Surg.* 2010;18(1):20–30.

Nauth A, McKee MD, Ristevski B, Hall J, Schemitsch EH. Distal humeral fractures in adults. *J Bone Joint Surg Am.* 2011;93(7): 686–700.

Humeral Shaft Fractures

chapter 24

CLASSIC ARTICLE

Authors: Sarmiento A, Kinman PB, Galvin EG, Schmitt RH, Phillips JG.

Title: Functional bracing of fractures of the shaft of the humerus.

Journal Information: *J Bone Joint Surg Am.* 1977;59:596–601.

Study Design: Retrospective Case Series

▸ 49 patients with 51 humeral shaft fractures treated with functional bracing.

▸ 13 open fractures, 38 closed fractures.

▸ Fracture location

  ▷ 9 proximal third

  ▷ 26 middle third

  ▷ 16 distal third

▸ Follow-up ranged from 2 to 30 months.

Results

▸ 98% union rate (1 nonunion in patient with metastatic breast cancer)

▸ 82% had full shoulder and elbow motion.

▸ 84% healed with less than 10 degrees of angular deformity.

▸ Varus deformity most common, average angulation 4 degrees of varus.

Conclusions

▶ The authors stated that their experience during the past 13 years with functional bracing for treatment of long bone fractures led them to assert that rigid immobilization of fracture fragments, adjacent joints, or both is not a necessary prerequisite for fracture healing.

▶ In contrast, it appeared that the motion that inevitably takes place at the fracture site when a brace is used enhances fracture healing.

▶ Firm compression of the soft tissues surrounding the fractured bone is applied by the rigid walls of the brace, and adequate alignment of the fragments is maintained with sufficient stability to permit uninterrupted osteogenesis.

Commentary

▶ Functional bracing provides a hydraulic compressive centripetal force that maintains fracture alignment.

▶ This landmark article provides a gold standard against which operative fixation has been judged.

▶ This study was performed prior to reliance on patient self-reported assessment and validated functional outcome scores.

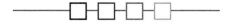

FEATURED ARTICLE

Authors: Sarmiento A, Horowitch A, Aboulafia A, Vangsness CT Jr.

Title: Functional bracing for comminuted extra-articular fractures of the distal third of the humerus.

Journal Information: *J Bone Joint Surg Br.* 1990;72(2):283–287.

Study Design: Retrospective Review

▶ Patients with extra-articular comminuted distal third humeral fractures treated with a prefabricated humeral fracture brace.

▶ 65 patients with clinical and radiographic records.

▸ 7 patients had radiographic records but not clinical records.

▸ Average age: 28 years (17 to 62 years), 37 males, 28 females.

▸ 11/65 (17%) open fractures (8 of these were gunshot wounds).

▸ Average time from injury to brace application: 12 days (4 to 45 days).

▸ 12/65 (18.5%) had an initial peripheral nerve injury

  ▷ 10 radial nerve palsies

  ▷ 2 radial nerve and partial median nerve palsies

Results

▸ 69/72 (96%) patients with radiographic records united.

▸ No reported infections.

▸ Nerve injuries

  ▷ 9/12 completely resolved at follow-up

  ▷ 3/12 had improving function at last follow-up visits of 2, 4, and 6 months

▸ Radiographic deformity

  ▷ 16% had no varus/valgus deformity

  ▷ 81% of patients had a varus deformity

    » Average varus deformity: 9 degrees

  ▷ 3% had a valgus deformity

▸ 36% had fracture site shortening

  ▷ Average shortening: 5 mm (2 to 15 mm)

▸ Movement limitations

  ▷ 45% had shoulder external rotation limitations with losses ranging from 5 to 45 degrees

  ▷ 15.5% had shoulder abduction limitations with losses ranging from 10 to 60 degrees

  ▷ 13% had shoulder flexion limitations with losses ranging from 5 to 20 degrees

  ▷ 26% had elbow flexion limitations with losses ranging from 5 to 25 degrees

  ▷ 24% had elbow extension limitations with losses ranging from 5 to 25 degrees

Conclusions

▸ The authors concluded that a prefabricated fracture brace provides satisfactory results for comminuted extra-articular distal-third humerus fractures.

> They also noted the high rate of nerve recovery and indicated that early exploration of nerve injury is not justified.

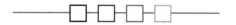

FEATURED ARTICLE

Authors: Dabezies EJ, Banta CJ II, Murphy CP, d'Ambrosia RD.

Title: Plate fixation of the humeral shaft for acute fractures, with and without radial nerve injuries.

Journal Information: *J Orthop Trauma*. 1992;6(1):10–13.

This is one of the top 20 cited papers published in the *Journal of Orthopaedic Trauma*, 1987 to 2007.

Study Design: Retrospective Review

> 44 consecutive acute humeral shaft fractures treated by ORIF.
> 15 radial nerve injuries were associated with the fractures.

Results

> 97% (43/44) healed at an average of 12 weeks.
> 1 fixation failure treated by revision with a longer plate and bone grafting, which subsequently healed.
> ROM of the shoulder and elbow were essentially normal.
> 8/9 fractures treated with 3.5-mm compression plates healed uneventfully.
> All 11 open fractures (8 from bullet wounds) healed uneventfully after early plating.
> Results of 15 radial nerve injuries
>> 12 anatomically intact radial nerve palsies recovered in 17 weeks on average after plate fixation
>> 1 lacerated nerve was sutured and recovered

▷ 1 nerve with segmental loss associated with an open fracture was left unrepaired

▷ 1 avulsed nerve associated with a closed fracture was left unrepaired

Conclusions

▸ The dissection required for plate fixation provides information that may be helpful in determining appropriate treatment of radial nerve injuries and the prognosis for spontaneous return of function when the nerve is found to be intact.

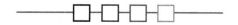

FEATURED ARTICLE

Authors: Chapman JR, Henley MB, Agel J, Benca PJ.

Title: Randomized prospective study of humeral shaft fracture fixation: intramedullary nails versus plates.

Journal Information: *J Orthop Trauma.* 2000;14(3):162–166.

Study Design: Prospective Randomization (Sealed-Envelope Technique)

▸ 84 patients with humeral shaft fractures (defined as being at least 3 cm distal to the surgical neck and at least 5 cm proximal to the olecranon fossa)

▷ 38 randomized to IM nail (antegrade)

▷ 46 randomized to plate fixation (4.5-mm dynamic compression and limited contact dynamic compression plates)

▸ Outcome measures

▷ Fracture healing

▷ Radial nerve recovery

▷ Infection

▷ Elbow and shoulder discomfort

- Radiographic measurements
  - ▷ Fracture alignment
  - ▷ Time to healing
  - ▷ Delayed union
  - ▷ Nonunion

Results

- Average follow-up: 13 months.
- No significant difference in healing rate ($P = .70$)
  - ▷ 42/46 (91%) of plate group were healed by 16 weeks
  - ▷ 33/38 (87%) of IM nail group healed by 16 weeks
- Significant association of shoulder pain with IM nail group ($P = .007$).
- Significant association of decreased shoulder motion with IM nail group ($P = .007$).
- Significant association of decreased elbow motion with plate group ($P = .03$), especially for distal-third shaft fractures.
- No significant association of elbow pain with plate group ($P = .123$).
- Nearly equal number of other complications in both groups.

Conclusions

- IM nailing and compression plate fixation are both predictable methods for achieving fracture stabilization and ultimate healing.
- Antegrade IM humeral nailing associated with shoulder pain and decreased shoulder motion.
- Plate fixation associated with decreased elbow motion.

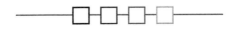

FEATURED ARTICLE

Authors: McCormack RG, Brien D, Buckley RE, McKee MD, Powell J, Schemitsch EH.

Title: Fixation of fractures of the shaft of the humerus by dynamic compression plate or intramedullary nail: a prospective randomized trial.

Journal Information: *J Bone Joint Surg Br.* 2000;82(3):337–339.

Study Design: Prospective, Multicenter (3 Canadian Tertiary-Care Centers) Randomized Study

- ▶ 44 patients with humeral shaft fractures randomized to the following:
  - ▷ ORIF with a dynamic compression plate
  - ▷ IM nail
    - » Initially antegrade but during the study changed to allow retrograde based on reports from other studies noting shoulder pain with antegrade nailing
- ▶ Minimum 6 months follow-up.
- ▶ Outcome measurements
  - ▷ American Shoulder and Elbow Surgeons (ASES) Score
  - ▷ VAS Pain Score
  - ▷ ROM
  - ▷ Time to return to normal activity

Results

- ▶ No significant differences in the function of the shoulder and elbow, as determined by the ASES Score, the VAS Pain Score, ROM, or the time taken to return to normal activity.
- ▶ Shoulder impingement
  - ▷ 1 in plate ORIF group
  - ▷ 6 in IM nail group (5 after antegrade insertion, 1 after retrograde insertion)
- ▶ Complications
  - ▷ 3 in plate ORIF group
    - » 1 nonunion, 1 intraoperative comminution, 1 minimal loss of fixation
  - ▷ 13 in IM nail group
    - » 3 iatrogenic nerve palsies, 1 late fracture, 2 nonunions, 2 intraoperative comminution, 1 infection, 3 severe shoulder impingement, 1 adhesive capsulitis
- ▶ Significantly more secondary surgeries in IM nail group ($P = .016$)
  - ▷ 1 in plate ORIF group
  - ▷ 7 in IM nail group

Conclusions

- ▶ The authors suggested that ORIF with a dynamic compression plate remains the best treatment for unstable fractures of the shaft of the humerus.

▸ IM nail fixation may be indicated for specific situations but is technically more demanding and has a higher rate of complications.

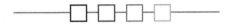

FEATURED ARTICLE

Authors: Tingstad EM, Wolinsky PR, Shyr Y, Johnson KD.

Title: Effect of immediate weightbearing on plated fractures of the humeral shaft.

Journal Information: *J Trauma.* 2000;49(2):278–280.

Study Design: Retrospective Review

▸ 83 humeral shaft fractures in 82 patients.

▸ All treated with ORIF using dynamic compression plate (nonlocked plate).

▸ Average age: 49 years (13 to 79 years), 44 males, 38 females.

▸ Postop weightbearing status of the involved humerus was based on the presence or absence of a lower extremity injury that required restricted weightbearing.

▸ Patients with associated injuries necessitating lower extremity nonweightbearing were allowed to bear weight through their plated humerus

  ▷ A patient who could not bear weight on 1 lower extremity was allowed to ambulate using crutches or a walker, fully weightbearing through both upper extremities

  ▷ A patient who could not bear weight on either lower extremity was allowed to transfer using the involved upper extremity

▸ Patients without associated lower extremity injuries were assumed to be nonweightbearing through their humerus.

▸ Based on these criteria

  ▷ 52% of the fractures were allowed to immediately bear full weight

  ▷ 40% were nonweightbearing

  ▷ 8% were cleared for transfers

Results

▸ 94% of fractures healed after the initial operation.

▸ Statistical analysis showed no relationship between weightbearing status and union rate.

▸ Secondary surgery to achieve union was required in 5 patients

▷ 2/33 (6%) patients in nonweightbearing group

▷ 3/50 (6%) patients in weightbearing group

▸ 1 hardware failure in each group.

▸ Radiographic alignment did not differ between the 2 groups.

Conclusions

▸ When indicated, immediate weightbearing following ORIF of humeral diaphyseal fractures is safe and efficacious.

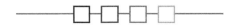

FEATURED ARTICLE

Authors: Oh CW, Byun YS, Oh JK, et al.

Title: Plating of humeral shaft fractures: comparison of standard conventional plating versus minimally invasive plating.

Journal Information: *Orthop Traumatol Surg Res.* 2012;98(1): 54–60.

Study Design: Retrospective Cohort Study

▸ Treatment differed during 2 time periods

1. 30 patients whose humeral shaft fractures were treated with ORIF from January 2003 to February 2006

2. 29 patients whose humeral shaft fractures were treated with minimally invasive plate osteosynthesis (MIPO) from March 2006 to April 2009

- Outcome measurements
  - ▷ UCLA Shoulder Score
  - ▷ Mayo Elbow Performance Index Score
  - ▷ Radiographic evaluation
  - ▷ Complications
- MIPO surgical technique
  - ▷ 4 to 5 cm distal anterior incision proximal to elbow crease
  - ▷ Sensory branch of musculocutaneous nerve protected after retracting the biceps muscle
  - ▷ Brachialis muscle split by blunt dissection
  - ▷ Submuscular tunnel developed using a 9- to 12-hole locking plate with an attached locking sleeve that served as a handle
  - ▷ Reduction achieved with manual traction
  - ▷ Plate fixed to anterior surface with 3 bicortical screws above and below the fracture
  - ▷ No exploration of the radial nerve

Results

- Significantly shorter operative time with MIPO ($P < .05$)
  - ▷ Average operative time for ORIF: 169 minutes
  - ▷ Average operative time for MIPO: 110 minutes
- No difference in time to union
  - ▷ Average 16.7 weeks in ORIF group
  - ▷ Average 17.3 weeks in MIPO group
- No difference in functional outcome scores
  - ▷ UCLA Shoulder Score
    - » Average 33.8 points in ORIF group
    - » Average 34.3 points in MIPO group
  - ▷ Mayo Elbow Score
    - » Average 97 points in ORIF group
    - » Average 97.6 points in MIPO group

- Complications
  - ▷ Nonunions: 3 in ORIF group, 1 in MIPO group
  - ▷ Postop radial nerve palsy: 1 in ORIF group, 1 in MIPO group
  - ▷ Deep infection: 1 in ORIF group, zero in MIPO group
  - ▷ Screw loosening: zero in ORIF group, 1 in MIPO group

Conclusions

- Minimally invasive plate osteosynthesis achieves results comparable to ORIF.

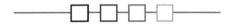

REVIEW ARTICLES

Gregory PR, Sanders RW. Compression plating versus intramedullary fixation of humeral shaft fractures. *J Am Acad Orthop Surg.* 1997;5(4):215–223.

Sarmiento A, Latta LL. Functional fracture bracing. *J Am Acad Orthop Surg.* 1999;7(1):66–75.

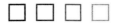

Proximal Humerus Fractures

chapter *25*

CLASSIC ARTICLE

Author: Neer CS II.

Title: Displaced proximal humeral fractures. I. Classification and evaluation.

Journal Information: *J Bone Joint Surg Am.* 1970;52(6): 1077–1089.

Study Design: Retrospective Review

▶ 300 displaced proximal humeral fractures and fracture-dislocations selected at random from those treated by closed reduction or surgery between 1953 and 1967

▷ Average age: 55.6 years (22 to 89 years)

▷ 162 closed reductions

▷ 75 open reductions

▷ 5 humeral head resections

▷ 63 prosthetic replacements

▶ X-rays prior to treatment were studied and the relationships of the major segments charted.

▶ Operative findings and photographs were correlated with x-ray findings.

Hak DJ.
Rapid Reference Review in Orthopedic Trauma:
Pivotal Papers Revealed (pp 253-263).
© 2013 SLACK Incorporated.

Conclusions

▸ Developed a classification based on the presence or absence of displacement of 1 or more of 4 major segments (articular surface of the humeral head, greater tuberosity, lesser tuberosity, and shaft).

▸ Defined displacement as > 1 cm or angulation > 45 degrees.

▸ Numerous studies both before and after this article have shown a low level of interobserver reliability for a wide range of classification systems.

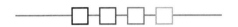

FEATURED ARTICLE

Authors: Sidor ML, Zuckerman JD, Lyon T, Koval K, Cuomo F, Schoenberg N.

Title: The Neer classification system for proximal humeral fractures: an assessment of interobserver reliability and intraobserver reproducibility.

Journal Information: *J Bone Joint Surg Am.* 1993;75(12):1745–1750.

Study Design: Radiographic Evaluation for Interobserver Reliability and Intraobserver Reproducibility

▸ X-rays of 50 proximal humerus fractures were reviewed and classified using the Neer classification system.

▸ Neer classification system
  ▹ Most widely used system to classify proximal humerus fractures
  ▹ 16-category system
  ▹ Based on the number and location of displaced fractures

▸ Shoulder trauma series reviewed
  ▹ Scapular AP
  ▹ Scapular lateral
  ▹ Axillary view

- Fracture classification assessed by 5 people
  ▷ Orthopedic shoulder specialist
  ▷ Orthopedic traumatologist
  ▷ Skeletal radiologist
  ▷ Fifth year orthopedic resident
  ▷ Second year orthopedic resident
  ▷ X-rays reviewed on 2 separate occasions 6 months apart
- Interobserver reliability assessed by comparing the classification determined by the 5 observers.
- Intraobserver reproducibility evaluated by comparison of each observer's first and second viewing.
- Calculated kappa (κ) reliability coefficients.

Results

- All 5 observers agreed on the classification for only 32% of cases in first viewing, and in only 30% in second viewing.
- Average interobserver reliability between paired observers: 0.52 (0.37 to 0.62).
- Average reproducibility was 0.66 and ranged from 0.83 for the shoulder specialist to 0.50 for the skeletal radiologist.

Commentary

- Many fracture classifications have relatively low interoberserver reliability and intraobserver reproducibility.

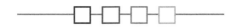

FEATURED ARTICLE

Authors: Jaberg H, Warner JJ, Jakob RP.

Title: Percutaneous stabilization of unstable fractures of the humerus.

Journal Information: *J Bone Joint Surg Am.* 1992;74(4):508–515.

Figure 25-1. Schematic diagram of recommended position of percutaneous fixation pins. 2 pins (a) are inserted from the lateral shaft. A third pin (b) is inserted from the anterior cortex. For cases with displaced greater tuberosity fractures, 2 pins (c) are also added.

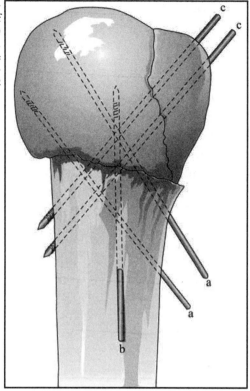

Study Design: Retrospective Review

▸ 48 proximal humerus fractures in 45 patients treated by closed reduction and percutaneous pinning using terminally threaded 2.5-mm wires (Figure 25-1).

▸ Average follow-up: 3 years (2 to 7 years).

▸ Average age: 63 years (17 to 85 years), 11 males, 37 females.

▸ Fracture pattern

▷ 29 2-part surgical neck

▷ 3 2-part anatomic neck

▷ 8 3-part proximal humerus fractures

▷ 5 4-part proximal humerus fractures

▷ 3 anterior fracture-dislocations

Fixation Technique

▸ 2 pins inserted in the lateral cortex just above the deltoid insertion and directed superiorly.

▸ 1 pin is inserted from anterior cortex and directed into humeral head.

▸ If greater tuberosity is displaced, it is reduced and fixed with 2 pins inserted into the fragment and directed inferiorly to engage the medial cortex.

▸ Pins should be widely spaced in the fracture fragments.

▸ Greater tuberosity pins are removed at 3 weeks.

▸ Remaining pins are removed at 6 weeks.

▸ Assessment: 18-point scale of Saillant and colleagues

  ▷ 0 to 3 points on 6 categories

  ▷ Pain

  ▷ Glenohumeral abduction

  ▷ Glenohumeral rotation at 0 degrees abduction

  ▷ Glenohumeral rotation at 90 degrees abduction

  ▷ Patient-subjective results

  ▷ Physician-subjective results

Results

▸ 34 (70%) good or excellent

▸ 10 (20%) fair

▸ 4 (8%) poor

▸ Complications

  ▷ 4 patients had a loss of fixation requiring repeat pinning

  ▷ 1 malunion

  ▷ 4 superficial pin tract infections

  ▷ 1 deep infection

  ▷ 2 nonunions

  ▷ 2 complete avascular necrosis (AVN) with collapse of humeral head

  ▷ 8 localized AVN with transient cyst formation and sclerosis that resolved over 1 to 2 years

Conclusions

▸ Percutaneous pinning is technically demanding.

▸ Results are comparable with or superior to previously described ORIF methods.

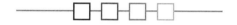

FEATURED ARTICLE

Authors: Olerud P, Ahrengart L, Ponzer S, Saving J, Tidermark J.

Title: Hemiarthroplasty versus nonoperative treatment of displaced 4-part proximal humeral fractures in elderly patients: a randomized controlled trial.

Journal Information: *J Shoulder Elbow Surg.* 2011;20(7): 1025–1033.

Study Design: Prospective Randomized Study (by Opaque Sealed Envelope)

▸ 55 elderly patients (age > 55 years) with displaced 4-part proximal humerus fractures

▷ 26 underwent hemiarthroplasty

≫ 1 additional patient was randomized to hemiarthroplasty but was treated with a locking plate

▷ 28 underwent nonoperative treatment

▸ Average age: 77 years (58 to 92 years), 8 males, 47 females.

▸ Follow-up

▷ 26 patients in hemiarthroplasty group and 25 patients in nonoperative group completed 12 months follow-up

▷ 24 patients in hemiarthroplasty group and 25 patients in nonoperative group completed 24 months follow-up

- Outcome measurements
  - ▷ VAS Pain Score
  - ▷ Constant Score
  - ▷ Disabilities of the Arm, Shoulder, and Hand (DASH) Score
  - ▷ Health-related quality of life (HRQoL) according to the Euro quality of life-5 dimensions (EQ-5D)

Results

- HRQoL EQ-5D (index) Score was significantly better in the hemiarthroplasty group at 2 years ($P = .02$)
  - ▷ Hemiarthroplasty group: 0.81
  - ▷ Nonoperative group: 0.65
- Average Pain Score better in hemiarthroplasty group at 2 years but difference not statistically significant ($P = .17$)
  - ▷ Hemiarthroplasty group: 15
  - ▷ Nonoperative group: 25
- Average DASH Score better in hemiarthroplasty group at 2 years but difference not statistically significant ($P = .25$)
  - ▷ Hemiarthroplasty group: 30
  - ▷ Nonoperative group: 37
- No significant difference in Constant Score.
- No significant difference in ROM
  - ▷ Both groups achieved an average flexion of 90 to 95 degrees and an average abduction of 85 to 90 degrees
- Additional surgery
  - ▷ 3 patients in the hemiarthroplasty group
  - ▷ 1 patient in the nonoperative group

Conclusions

- Hemiarthroplasty was associated with a significant advantage in quality of life, compared to nonoperative treatment of displaced 4-part proximal humerus fractures.
- The main advantage of hemiarthroplasty appears to be less pain.
- No difference in ROM between hemiarthroplasty and nonoperative treatment.

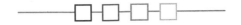

FEATURED ARTICLE

Authors: Olerud P, Ahrengart L, Ponzer S, Saving J, Tidermark J.

Title: Internal fixation versus nonoperative treatment of displaced 3-part proximal humeral fractures in elderly patients: a randomized controlled trial.

Journal Information: *J Shoulder Elbow Surg.* 2011;20(5):747–755.

Study Design: Prospective Randomized (by Opaque Sealed Envelope) Study

- 59 displaced 3-part fractures of the proximal humerus in elderly (> 55 years) patients
  - 29 underwent ORIF with a locking plate
  - 29 underwent nonoperative treatment
  - 1 patient randomized to ORIF was treated with hemiarthroplasty
- Average age: 74 years (56 to 92 years), 12 males, 47 females.
- Follow-up
  - 27 patients in each group completed 12 months follow-up
  - 27 patients in ORIF group and 26 patients in nonoperative group completed 24 months follow-up
- Outcome measurements
  - Constant Score
  - DASH Score
  - HRQoL according to the EQ-5D

Results

- At 2-year follow-up, ROM, function, and HRQoL were all better in the locking plate group, but given the small sample size, none of these differences were statistically significant.
- ROM at 2 years
  - Average forward flexion not statistically different (*P* = .36)
    - » Locking plate group: 120 degrees
    - » Nonoperative group: 111 degrees

- ▷ Average abduction not statistically different (*P* = .28)
  - » Locking plate group: 114 degrees
  - » Nonoperative group: 106 degrees
- ▶ Constant Score not statistically different (*P* = .19)
  - ▷ Locking plate group: 61
  - ▷ Nonoperative group: 58
- ▶ DASH Score not statistically different
  - ▷ Locking plate group: 26
  - ▷ Nonoperative group: 35
- ▶ Average EQ-5D (index) Score not statistically different (*P* = .26)
  - ▷ Locking plate group: 0.70
  - ▷ Nonoperative group: 0.59
- ▶ Good initial reduction in 86% of locking plate ORIF
  - ▷ 13% (4/29) in ORIF group had a fracture complication requiring major reoperation
    - » 1 primary infection
    - » 1 hematogenous infection
    - » 1 nonunion
    - » 1 severe AVN
  - ▷ 17% (5/29) in ORIF group had a minor reoperation (hardware removal and release of adhesions performed between 1 and 2 years postop)
    - » 1 for screw penetration
    - » 2 for postop stiffness
    - » 2 for impingement
  - ▷ 17% (5/29) had evidence of screw penetration on postop x-ray
  - ▷ 3 additional patients showed screw penetration at 4 months follow-up
- ▶ One nonunion in nonoperative group.

Conclusions

- ▶ The authors concluded that ORIF with a locking plate was better than nonoperative treatment.
- ▶ However, additional surgery was required in 30% of patients treated with ORIF.

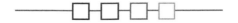

FEATURED ARTICLE

Authors: Südkamp N, Bayer J, Hepp P, et al.

Title: Open reduction and internal fixation of proximal humeral fractures with use of the locking proximal humerus plate. Results of a prospective, multicenter, observational study.

Journal Information: *J Bone Joint Surg Am.* 2009;91(6): 1320–1328.

Study Design: Prospective, Multicenter, Observational Study

▸ 187 patients with proximal humeral fracture treated by ORIF using a locking proximal humeral plate.

▸ Designed to evaluate functional outcome and complication rate.

▸ Average age: 63 years, 52 males, 135 females.

▸ Outcome measurements

  ▷ Pain

  ▷ Shoulder ROM

  ▷ Strength

  ▷ Constant Score

  ▷ DASH Score

▸ Follow-up

  ▷ 88% (165 patients) completed 3-month follow-up

  ▷ 84% (158 patients) completed 6-month follow-up

  ▷ 83% (155 patients) completed 1-year follow-up

Results

▸ Average ROM and average Constant Score substantially improved between 3 months, 6 months, and 1 year postop.

▸ Average Constant Score at 1 year

  ▷ Injured side 70.6 ± 13.7 points

  ▷ Uninjured side to 85.1% ± 14.0%

▸ Average DASH Score at 1 year

  ▷ 15.2 ± 16.8 points

- Complications
  - ▷ 34% (52/155) of patients at 1-year follow-up had experienced 62 complications
  - ▷ 40% (25/62) of complications were related to incorrect surgical technique and were present at the end of the operative procedure
  - ▷ Intraoperative screw perforation of the humeral head was the most common complication
    - » 14% (21/155) incidence of intraoperative screw penetration
  - ▷ 29 patients (19%) had an unplanned second operation within 1 year

Conclusions

- Treatment of proximal humeral fractures with a locking plate can lead to a good functional outcome.
- Many complications are related to improper surgical technique (iatrogenic errors).
- The authors recommended a careful final fluoroscopic evaluation with rotation of the humeral head to verify correct screw placement.

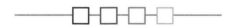

REVIEW ARTICLES

Cadet ER, Ahmad CS. Hemiarthroplasty for three- and four-part proximal humerus fractures. *J Am Acad Orthop Surg.* 2012;20(1):17–27.

George MS. Fractures of the greater tuberosity of the humerus. *J Am Acad Orthop Surg.* 2007;15(10):607–613.

Naranja RJ Jr, Iannotti JP. Displaced three- and four-part proximal humerus fractures: evaluation and management. *J Am Acad Orthop Surg.* 2000;8(6):373–382.

Nho SJ, Brophy RH, Barker JU, Cornell CN, MacGillivray JD. Innovations in the management of displaced proximal humerus fractures. *J Am Acad Orthop Surg.* 2007;15(1):12–26.

Ricchetti ET, DeMola PM, Roman D, Abboud JA. The use of precontoured humeral locking plates in the management of displaced proximal humerus fracture. *J Am Acad Orthop Surg.* 2009;17(9):582–590.

Scapula and Glenoid Fractures

chapter **26**

CLASSIC ARTICLE
Author: Goss TP.
Title: Double disruptions of the superior shoulder suspensory complex.
Journal Information: *J Orthop Trauma.* 1993;7(2):99–106.

Study Design: Review Article With Representative Clinical Cases

▶ Introduced the "double-disruption" concept of injury to the superior shoulder suspensory complex.

▶ Superior shoulder suspensory complex (Figure 26-1)

  ▷ Bone/soft-tissue ring at the end of a superior and inferior bone strut that is composed of the following:

   » Glenoid process

   » Coracoid process

   » Coracoclavicular (CC) ligaments

   » Distal clavicle

   » Acromioclavicular (AC) joint

   » Acromial process

Hak DJ.
*Rapid Reference Review in Orthopedic Trauma:
Pivotal Papers Revealed (pp 265-270).*
© 2013 SLACK Incorporated.

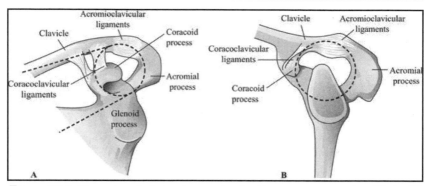

Figure 26-1. Illustrations depicting the superior shoulder suspensory complex. (A) An AP view of the bony/soft-tissue ring and superior/inferior bony struts. (B) A lateral view of the bony/soft-tissue ring.

▷ Maintains a normal stable relationship between the scapula/upper extremity and the axial skeleton, allows limited motion at the AC joint and CC ligaments, and provides a firm attachment point for several soft-tissue structures

▶ Traumatic disruptions of 1 of the components are common and tend to be minor injuries that do not significantly compromise the overall integrity of the complex.

▶ If the traumatic force is sufficiently severe or adversely directed, the ring may fail in 2 or more places (a double disruption), resulting in significant displacement and an unstable anatomic situation, leading to adverse long-term healing and functional consequences.

▶ The double disruption may consist of the following:

  ▷ 2 torn ligaments

  ▷ 2 fractures

  ▷ 1 fracture and 1 torn ligament

▶ If displacement is unacceptable, surgical reduction and stabilization of 1 or more of the sites is necessary.

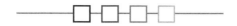

FEATURED ARTICLE

Authors: Zlowodzki M, Bhandari M, Zelle BA, Kregor PJ, Cole PA.

Title: Treatment of scapula fractures: systematic review of 520 fractures in 22 case series.

Journal Information: *J Orthop Trauma.* 2006;20(3):230–233.

Study Design: Systematic Review

▶ 22 case studies of scapula fractures.

▶ Criteria for inclusion of studies

  ▷ More than 5 scapular fractures

  ▷ Reported categorical functional results (eg, excellent, good, fair, poor)

  ▷ Reported a combination of pain assessment and ROM

▶ Study's objectives

  ▷ Determine incidence of operative and nonoperative treatment of different scapular fractures

  ▷ Systematically stratify the reported results of operatively and nonoperatively treated scapula fractures and summarize functional results

  ▷ Quantify infection and secondary surgical procedure rates after operative treatment

▶ Scapula fracture background statistics

  ▷ Represent 3% to 5% of all fractures of the shoulder girdle

  ▷ Make up < 1% of all fractures

  ▷ Typically occur as a result of high-energy trauma

  ▷ 90% of patients have associated injuries

Results

▶ 80% of all fractures with glenoid involvement were treated operatively.

▶ Operative treatment of glenoid fractures resulted in excellent or good outcomes in 82% of cases.

▶ 99% of isolated scapula body fractures were treated nonoperatively.

▶ Nonoperative treatment of isolated scapular body fractures resulted in excellent or good results in 86% of cases.

- ► 83% of scapular neck fractures with intact glenoid were treated nonoperatively.
- ► Nonoperative treatment of isolated scapular neck fractures resulted in excellent or good results in 77% of cases.
- ► In a smaller subset, nonoperative treatment of scapular neck with associated clavicle fractures resulted in excellent or good results in 94% of cases.
- ► Deep infection rate in operative cases: 1.4% (2/141).
- ► Superficial infection rate in operative cases: 2.1% (3/141).
- ► 23 secondary surgical procedures (16.5%) reported after operative treatment
  - ▷ 8 manipulations
  - ▷ 7 hardware removals
  - ▷ 3 irrigation and débridements
  - ▷ 2 hematoma evacuations
  - ▷ 2 revision ORIFs
  - ▷ 1 glenohumeral arthrodesis

Conclusions

- ► The authors cautioned that a valid comparison between operative and nonoperative treatment cannot be made for any fracture type due to the following:
  - ▷ Low number of scapular neck and body fractures treated operatively
  - ▷ Low number of glenoid fractures treated nonoperatively
  - ▷ High variability between studies
  - ▷ Different nonvalidated and nonspecific outcome measures
  - ▷ High incidence of associated injuries
  - ▷ Methodological limitations of many studies

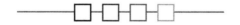

FEATURED ARTICLE

Authors: Anavian J, Gauger EM, Schroder LK, Wijdicks CA, Cole PA.

Title: Surgical and functional outcomes after operative management of complex and displaced intra-articular glenoid fractures.

Journal Information: *J Bone Joint Surg Am.* 2012;94(7):645–653.

Study Design: Prospective Cohort Study

▸ 33 displaced intra-articular glenoid fractures treated by ORIF between 2002 and 2009.

▸ Operative indication was the articular fracture gap or step-off of ≥ 4 mm.

▸ Average age: 44 years (18 to 75 years), 31 males, 2 females.

▸ Average follow-up: 27 months (12 to 73 months).

▸ Fracture configuration

  ▷ 2 had 4 articular fragments

  ▷ 16 had 3 articular fragments

  ▷ 15 had 2 articular fragments

  ▷ 25 patients also had extra-articular scapular involvement

▸ Surgical approach

  ▷ 21 posterior

  ▷ 7 anterior

  ▷ 5 combined anterior and posterior approaches

▸ Functional outcomes evaluated in 30/33 (91%) patients

  ▷ Disabilities of the Arm, Shoulder, and Hand (DASH)

  ▷ SF-36

  ▷ Shoulder motion and strength

  ▷ Return to work and/or activities

Results at Final Follow-Up

▸ All patients had radiographic union.

▸ Average DASH: 10.8 (0 to 42).

- All average SF-36 subscores comparable with those of the normal population.
- 26/30 patients (87%) were pain free.
- 4 patients had mild pain with prolonged activity.
- 27/30 patients (90%) returned to their preinjury level of work and/or activities.
- Complications
  - ▷ 1 intra-articular screw requiring repeat surgery
  - ▷ 1 postop stiffness requiring manipulation
  - ▷ 1 symptomatic ectopic bone requiring surgical resection

Conclusions

- Surgical treatment for complex, displaced intra-articular glenoid fractures with or without involvement of the scapular neck and body can be associated with good functional outcomes and a low complication rate.

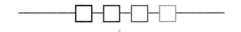

REVIEW ARTICLES

Cole PA, Gauger EM, Schroder LK. Management of scapular fractures. *J Am Acad Orthop Surg.* 2012;20(3):130–141.

DeFranco MJ, Patterson BM. The floating shoulder. *J Am Acad Orthop Surg.* 2006;148(8):499–509.

Goss TP. Scapular fractures and dislocations: diagnosis and treatment. *J Am Acad Orthop Surg.* 1995;3(1):22–33.

Lantry JM, Roberts CS, Giannoudis PV. Operative treatment of scapular fractures: a systematic review. *Injury.* 2008;39(3):271–283.

Lapner PC, Uhthoff HK, Papp S. Scapula fractures. *Orthop Clin North Am.* 2008;39(4):459–474.

Owens BD, Goss TP. The floating shoulder. *J Bone Joint Surg Br.* 2006; 88(11):1419–1424.

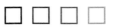

Clavicle Fractures

chapter 27

FEATURED ARTICLE

Author: Canadian Orthopaedic Trauma Society.

Title: Nonoperative treatment compared with plate fixation of displaced midshaft clavicular fractures. A multicenter, randomized clinical trial.

Journal Information: *J Bone Joint Surg Am.* 2007;89(1):1–10.

Study Design: Prospective, Multicenter, Randomized Clinical Trial Conducted at 8 Canadian Centers

▸ 132 patients (age 16 to 60 years) with displaced (no cortical contact between the main proximal and distal fragments) middle-third clavicle fractures were randomized to either plate fixation (67 patients) or nonoperative treatment with a sling (65 patients).

▸ Patient outcome measures
  ▷ Constant Shoulder Score
  ▷ Disabilities of the Arm, Shoulder, and Hand (DASH) score

▸ 1-year follow-up available for 111 patients (62 ORIF, 49 nonoperative).

Results

▸ Constant shoulder and DASH scores were significantly improved at all time points in the operative treatment group
  ▷ Magnitude of these differences was approximately 10 points, which is considered a clinically measurable amount

Hak DJ.
*Rapid Reference Review in Orthopedic Trauma:
Pivotal Papers Revealed (pp 271-277).*
© 2013 SLACK Incorporated.

- Average time to union
  - ▷ 16.4 weeks in operative group
  - ▷ 28.4 weeks in nonoperative group
- Statistically more nonunions in nonoperative treatment group (P = .042)
  - ▷ 2 nonunions in operative group
  - ▷ 7 nonunions in nonoperative group
- 9 symptomatic malunions in the nonoperative group, compared to 0 in operative group (P = .001).
- Significantly more complications in the nonoperative treatment group (P = .008)
  - ▷ 63% complication rate in nonoperative group
  - ▷ 37% complication rate in operative treatment group
- 9 hardware-related complications in the operative group included the following:
  - ▷ 5 symptomatic hardware requiring removal (the most common reason for repeat surgery in the operative treatment group)
  - ▷ 3 wound infections
  - ▷ 1 early mechanical failure
- At 1 year, patients in the operative group were more likely to be satisfied with their shoulder appearance (P = .001) and with their shoulder in general (P = .002).

Conclusions

- The investigators concluded that operative treatment of displaced clavicle fractures result in improved functional outcomes and a lower rate of malunion and nonunion.

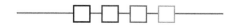

FEATURED ARTICLE

Authors: McKee RC, Whelan DB, Schemitsch EH, McKee MD.

Title: Operative versus nonoperative care of displaced midshaft clavicular fractures: a meta-analysis of randomized clinical trials.

Journal Information: *J Bone Joint Surg Am*. 2012;94(8):675–684.

Study Design: Systematic Literature Review

- 6 randomized clinical trials comparing operative versus nonoperative treatment of displaced midshaft clavicle fractures.
- 412 patients total
  - ▷ 200 nonoperative treatment
  - ▷ 212 operative treatment
    - » 3 studies used plate fixation
    - » 3 studies used IM fixation
- Study methodology evaluated using Detsky Quality Assessment Scale
  - ▷ Average Detsky score: 15.3 (14 to 16; one study was in abstract form and methodology could not be evaluated)
  - ▷ 14-item index that evaluates 5 categories of study design (maximum score 20 if positive study, 21 if negative study)
    - » Randomization
    - » 5 studies used sealed envelope technique, which is considered suboptimal by modern clinical trial standards
    - » Outcomes measures
    - » Eligibility criteria
    - » Interventions
    - » Statistics

Results

- Nonunion rate significantly higher following nonoperative treatment (29/200, 14.5%) than operative treatment (3/212, 1.4%; P = .001).
- Symptomatic malunion rate higher following nonoperative treatment (17/200, 8.5%) than operative treatment (0/212) (P < .001).

Conclusions

- Operative treatment had significantly lower rates of nonunion and symptomatic malunion and had an earlier functional return.
- Investigators cautioned that, at present, there is little evidence to show that the long-term functional outcome of operative treatment is significantly superior to nonoperative treatment.

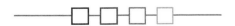

FEATURED ARTICLE

Authors: Smekal V, Irenberger A, Struve P, Wambacher M, Krappinger D, Kralinger FS.

Title: Elastic stable intramedullary nailing versus nonoperative treatment of displaced midshaft clavicular fractures—a randomized, controlled, clinical trial.

Journal Information: *J Orthop Trauma.* 2009;23(2):106–112.

Study Design: Prospective Randomized Study

- 68 adult patients with displaced midshaft clavicle fractures.
- Randomized to treatment with either of the following:
  - ▷ Elastic stable IM nailing (2.5-mm titanium endomedullary nail)
  - ▷ Nonoperative treatment with a sling
- 60 patients completed 2-year follow-up (30 operative, 30 nonoperative).
- Patient outcome measurements
  - ▷ Constant Shoulder Score
  - ▷ DASH Score

Results

- DASH Scores were improved in the operative group
  - ▷ These differences were statistically significant during the first 18 weeks
- Constant Shoulder Scores were significantly improved in the operative group after 6 months.
- Average time to union significantly shortened in operative treatment group ($P = .04$)
  - ▷ 12.1 weeks in operative group
  - ▷ 17.6 weeks in nonoperative group
- Nonunions
  - ▷ No nonunions in operative group
  - ▷ 3 nonunions in nonoperative group

- There were more complications in the nonoperative group, but this difference was not significant
  ▷ 10 complications in the operative group, including 2 implant failures and 1 delayed union
  ▷ 14 complications in the nonoperative group, including 6 delayed unions, 3 nonunions, and 2 symptomatic malunions
- Once the fracture was healed, implant removal was offered to all patients. Implant removal was performed in 25 cases, but reportedly only 2 patients were experiencing pain at the medial insertion site at the time of implant removal.

Conclusions

- The investigators concluded that treatment of displaced midshaft clavicle fractures with an elastic IM nail resulted in a lower rate of nonunion and delayed union, a faster return to daily activities, and a better functional outcome.

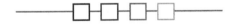

FEATURED ARTICLE

Authors: McKee MD, Pedersen EM, Jones C, et al.

Title: Deficits following nonoperative treatment of displaced midshaft clavicular fractures.

Journal Information: *J Bone Joint Surg Am.* 2006;88(1):35–40.

Study Design: Case Series

- Investigators used a patient-based outcome questionnaire and objective muscle strength testing to evaluate a series of patients who had received nonoperative care for a displaced midshaft fracture of the clavicle.
- Prior to this report, most investigators used radiographic and surgeon-based outcomes, reporting few functional deficits following nonoperative treatment.

- Studied 30 patients who had been treated nonoperatively for a displaced midshaft fracture of the clavicle.
- Average age: 37 years (19 to 67 years), 22 males, 8 females.
- This group came from a population of 107 adult patients treated for a displaced clavicle fracture between 1994 and 2000.
- Median time from injury: 55 months (12 to 72 months).
- Patient outcome measures
  ▷ Constant Shoulder Score
  ▷ DASH Score
- Objective shoulder muscle strength testing was performed with the Baltimore Therapeutic Equipment Work Simulator, with the uninjured arm serving as a control.

Results

- Good ROM with flexion averaging 170 ± 20 degrees and abduction averaging 165 ± 25 degrees.
- Compared with the strength of the uninjured shoulder, the strength of the injured shoulder was significantly reduced ($P < .05$ for all values)
  ▷ 81% for maximum flexion, 75% for endurance of flexion
  ▷ 82% for maximum abduction, 67% for endurance of abduction
  ▷ 81% for maximum external rotation, 82% for endurance of external rotation
  ▷ 85% for maximum internal rotation, 78% for endurance of internal rotation
- Patient outcome measures indicated substantial residual disability.
- Average Constant Shoulder Score was 71 points, compared with a published normative value for the general population of 92 points (lower Constant Shoulder Score indicates poorer function).
- Average DASH Score was 24.6 points, compared with a published normative value for the general population of 10.1 points (higher DASH Score indicates poorer function).

Conclusions

▸ The authors concluded that traditional surgeon-based methods of evaluation may be insensitive to loss of muscle strength.

▸ Using more objective measures, they found residual deficits in shoulder strength and endurance, which may be related to the significant level of dysfunction detected by the patient-based outcome measures.

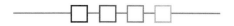

REVIEW ARTICLES

Jeray KJ. Acute midshaft clavicular fracture. *J Am Acad Orthop Surg.* 2007;15(4):239–248.

Khan LA, Bradnock TJ, Scott C, Robinson CM. Fractures of the clavicle. *J Bone Joint Surg Am.* 2009;91(2):447–460.

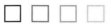

Compartment Syndrome

chapter 28

CLASSIC ARTICLE

Authors: Heckman MM, Whitesides TE Jr, Grewe SR, Rooks MD.

Title: Compartment pressure in association with closed tibial fractures. The relationship between tissue pressure, compartment, and the distance from the site of the fracture.

Journal Information: *J Bone Joint Surg Am.* 1994;76(9): 1285–1292.

Study Design: Prospective Cohort Study

▸ Studied 25 patients with closed tibial shaft fractures.

▸ Measured compartment pressures in all 4 compartments and at different locations in each compartment
  ▹ At the level of the fracture
  ▹ At 5-cm increments proximal and distal to the fracture
  ▹ Pressure measurements were repeated at 4-hour intervals or less until a safe peak pressure had been obtained and 2 consecutive measurements done 2 to 4 hours later had shown a gradual decrease in pressure to within a safe range

▸ They defined the safe range as a ΔP of 20 mm Hg (diastolic pressure minus compartment pressure).

Hak DJ.
Rapid Reference Review in Orthopedic Trauma: Pivotal Papers Revealed (pp 279-287).
© 2013 SLACK Incorporated.

Results

▸ Peak compartment pressures were usually found at the level of the fracture and were always within 5 cm of the fracture site.

▸ The measured pressure decreased steadily at increasing distances proximal and distal to the site of the highest recorded pressure.

▸ Decreases of 20 mm Hg 5 cm adjacent to the site of the peak pressure were common.

▸ The highest pressures were recorded in the anterior and the deep posterior compartments in 20 patients, including all 5 who underwent fasciotomy.

▸ Compartment syndrome was diagnosed based on clinical findings in 5 patients, and the diagnosis was confirmed by peak compartment pressures of more than the critical threshold (within 20 mm Hg of the diastolic blood pressure).

▸ 3 of these 5 patients had pressures less than the critical threshold within 5 cm of the site of the peak pressure.

Conclusions

▸ Failure to measure tissue pressure within a few centimeters of the zone of peak pressure may result in a serious underestimation of the maximum compartment pressure.

▸ They recommended that when compartment syndrome is clinically suspected, measurements should be performed in both the anterior and the deep posterior compartments at the level of the fracture, as well as at locations proximal and distal to the zone of the fracture to determine the highest tissue pressure.

▸ The highest pressure should be used in the decision-making process.

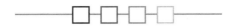

FEATURED ARTICLE

Authors: Matsen FA III, Winquist RA, Krugmire RB Jr.

Title: Diagnosis and management of compartmental syndromes.

Journal Information: *J Bone Joint Surg Am.* 1980;62(2):286–291.

▶ This article summarizes the signs and symptoms of compartment syndrome.

▶ It also includes diagrams showing the surgical technique for a single-incision lateral 4-compartment lower leg fasciotomy and for volar forearm fasciotomy.

Study Design: Prospective Cohort Study

▶ Evaluation of intracompartmental pressures using the infusion technique to evaluate 31 compartments in 30 patients

▷ 25 anterior tibial compartments

▷ 3 deep posterior tibial compartments

▷ 2 volar forearm compartments

▷ 1 anterior thigh compartment

▶ 13 patients had pressures > 30 mm Hg but did not undergo fasciotomy because of their benign clinical exam.

▶ All cases with pressures > 55 mm Hg displayed significant losses of neuromuscular function.

▶ They noted that individuals vary in their tolerance to increased pressures—there was a range of pressures in which some patients demonstrated neuromuscular deficits while others did not.

▶ They suggested that using a single critical pressure above which fasciotomy should be performed is of limited value

▷ If a low value is selected, there will be many unnecessary fasciotomies

▷ If a high value is selected, some patients who would benefit from fasciotomy may not undergo fasciotomy

Conclusions

▶ As a result of their clinical study, they recommended that > 45 mm Hg was a relative indication for fasciotomy, assuming a normal blood pressure.

▶ They went on to recommend that this indication must be tempered by the patient's overall condition and the trend of symptoms, signs, and pressure measurements.

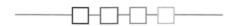

FEATURED ARTICLE

Authors: Mubarak SJ, Owen CA.

Title: Double-incision fasciotomy of the leg for decompression in compartment syndromes.

Journal Information: *J Bone Joint Surg Am.* 1977;59(2):184–187.

Study Design: Cadaveric Study

▶ This classic paper nicely describes the surgical technique for 2-incision fasciotomy of the lower leg (Figures 28-1 and 28-2).

▶ Anterolateral incision 2 cm anterior to fibular shaft

   » Superficial peroneal nerve is at risk in the distal third of the leg

   » Access to anterior and lateral compartment

  ▷ Posteromedial incision

   » Saphenous vein and nerve are at risk

   » Access to deep posterior and superficial posterior compartments

▶ Documented effectiveness of 2-incision fasciotomy in 3 cadaveric specimens in which saline was injected into the compartments until compartment pressures were 30 to 90 mm Hg

  ▷ Skin incisions alone only decreased compartment pressure by an average of 5 mm Hg

  ▷ Following double-incision fasciotomy, compartment pressures fell to normal levels

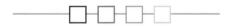

FEATURED ARTICLE

Authors: McQueen MM, Christie J, Court-Brown CM.

Title: Acute compartment syndrome in tibial diaphyseal fractures.

Journal Information: *J Bone Joint Surg Br.* 1996;78(1):95–98.

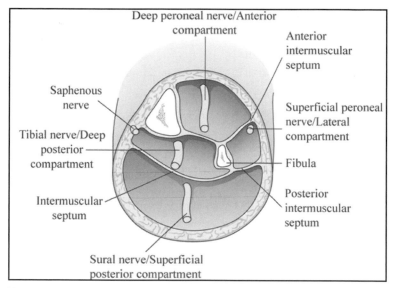

Figure 28-1. Compartments of the lower leg and their associated structures.

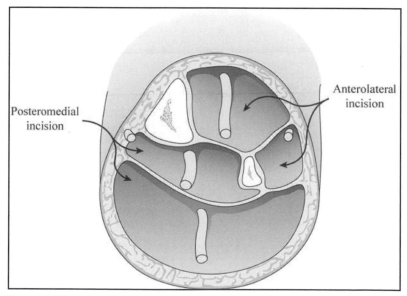

Figure 28-2. Diagram depicting a 2-incision fasciotomy of the lower leg.

Study Design: Retrospective Review

▶ 25 patients with tibial shaft fractures that had been complicated by compartment syndrome.

▶ Average age: 28 years (15 to 83 years), 23 males, 2 females.

▶ 23 closed fractures, 2 open fractures.

▶ Mechanism of injury
  ▷ 16 sporting injuries
  ▷ 7 road-traffic accidents
  ▷ 1 simple fall
  ▷ 1 fall from 30 feet

▶ 2 patients died from their injuries.

▶ Average follow-up of surviving patients: 10.5 months (4 to 32 months).

▶ 13 patients had continuous pressure monitoring of the anterior compartment using a slit catheter within 8 hours of injury.

▶ 12 cases did not have continuous monitoring
  ▷ 10 of these cases had pressure measurement to confirm the clinical diagnosis and compartment syndrome and underwent immediate fasciotomy
  ▷ 2 cases had no monitoring

Results

▶ The anterior compartment was involved in all 25 cases
  ▷ 12 cases had isolated involvement of the anterior compartment
  ▷ 6 cases had involvement of all 4 compartments
  ▷ 3 cases had involvement of anterior and lateral compartments
  ▷ 4 cases had involvement of anterior and deep posterior compartments

▶ Fasciotomy performed significantly earlier in the monitored group ($P < .05$)
  ▷ Average delay from injury to fasciotomy in the monitored group was 16 hours
  ▷ Average delay from injury to fasciotomy in the nonmonitored group was 32 hours

▶ Outcome
  ▷ The nonmonitored group had a significantly higher rate of sequelae ($P < .01$)
  ▷ Of the 12 surviving patients in the monitored group, none had any sequelae of compartment syndrome
  ▷ Of the 11 surviving patients in the nonmonitored group, 10 had definite sequelae with muscle weakness and contractures

- Time to radiographic union
  - ▷ Bone union in the nonmonitored fractures was significantly delayed ($P < .05$), suggesting that muscle necrosis may have impaired extraosseous blood flow leading to impaired healing
  - ▷ Average time to union in monitored fractures: 17 weeks (9 to 26 weeks)
  - ▷ Average time to union in nonmonitored fractures: 25 weeks (13 to 42 weeks)
  - ▷ There were no delayed unions in the monitored group, but 3 fractures in the nonmonitored group required additional surgery to achieve union

Conclusions

- The authors recommended that, when equipment is available, all patients with tibial fractures should have continuous pressure monitoring of the anterior compartment.

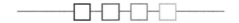

FEATURED ARTICLE

Authors: McQueen MM, Court-Brown CM.

Title: Compartment monitoring in tibial fractures. The pressure threshold for decompression.

Journal Information: *J Bone Joint Surg Br.* 1996;78(1):99–104.

Study Design: Prospective Study

- 116 patients with tibial diaphyseal fractures.
- This paper popularized the concept of ΔP = diastolic pressure minus compartment pressure.
- Average age: 33 years (14 to 85 years), 92 males and 24 females.
- Mechanism of injury
  - ▷ 42 sports injuries
  - ▷ 39 road traffic accidents
  - ▷ 29 falls
  - ▷ 6 other

- 16 open fractures, 100 closed fractures.
- Treatment
  - ▷ 90 IM nail
  - ▷ 15 external fixation
  - ▷ 7 casts
  - ▷ 4 plate fixation
  - ▷ 72 patients underwent operations within 24 hours of injury
- Average follow-up: 15 months (6 to 59 months).
- Continuous anterior compartment pressure monitoring was performed perioperatively and for 24 hours postop, or longer if indicated, using a slit catheter.

Results

- 3 patients (2.6%) had acute compartment syndrome.
- Elevated compartment pressures seen in first 12 hours
  - ▷ Average compartment pressure: 30 mm Hg (5 to 55)
  - ▷ 53 patients had pressures higher than 30 mm Hg
  - ▷ 30 patients had pressures higher than 40 mm Hg
  - ▷ 4 patients had pressures higher than 50 mm Hg
  - ▷ 1 patient had a ΔP less than 30 mm Hg, and he underwent fasciotomy
  - ▷ In 6 patients, the average ΔP was 30 mm Hg for the first 12 hours, but in all of them the absolute pressure fell, and the ΔP increased over the second 12 hours. None had any sequelae
- Elevated compartment pressures seen between 12 and 24 hours
  - ▷ Average compartment pressure: 25 mm Hg (5 to 75)
  - ▷ 28 patients had pressures higher than 30 mm Hg
  - ▷ 7 patients had pressures higher than 40 mm Hg
  - ▷ 2 patients had absolute pressures of higher than 50 mm Hg, and both had a ΔP less than 30 mm Hg in the second 12 hours and underwent fasciotomy
- No patients had any sequelae of compartment syndrome at their latest follow-up.
- Had they used 30 mm Hg absolute pressure as the threshold for fasciotomy, as recommended by several authors, then 53 patients would have had a fasciotomy.

▸ Because only 3 fasciotomies were performed, using this threshold would have led to 50 (43%) unnecessary fasciotomies.

▸ Had they used 40 mm Hg absolute pressure, then 27 patients (23%) would have had an unnecessary fasciotomy.

Conclusions

▸ Absolute compartment pressure is an unreliable indication of the need for fasciotomy.

▸ The use of a differential pressure (ΔP) of 30 mm Hg as a threshold for fasciotomy led to no missed cases of acute compartment syndrome.

▸ The authors recommended that fasciotomy should be performed if the differential pressure (ΔP) level drops to under 30 mm Hg.

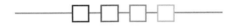

REVIEW ARTICLES

Olson SA, Glasgow RR. Acute compartment syndrome in lower extremity musculoskeletal trauma. *J Am Acad Orthop Surg.* 2005;13(7):436–444.

Prasarn ML, Ouellette EA. Acute compartment syndrome of the upper extremity. *J Am Acad Orthop Surg.* 2011;19(1):49–58.

Whitesides TE, Heckman MM. Acute compartment syndrome: update on diagnosis and treatment. *J Am Acad Orthop Surg.* 1996;4(4):209–218.

Polytrauma

chapter 29

CLASSIC ARTICLE

Authors: Bone LB, McNamara K, Shine B, Border J.

Title: Mortality in multiple trauma patients with fractures.

Journal Information: *J Trauma*. 1994;37(2):262–264.

This is one of the top 20 cited papers published in the *Journal of Orthopaedic Trauma*, 1987 to 2007.

Study Design: Retrospective, Multicenter (6 North American Sites) Study

▸ Examined mortality rate of multiply injured patients who had early total care of their fractures (ORIF within 48 hours of injury).
▸ Inclusion criteria
  ▷ Injury Severity Score (ISS) ≥ 18
  ▷ At least 1 fracture involving either
    » Femur
    » Pelvis or acetabulum
    » Bilateral tibial fractures
    » 1 tibia fracture along with another fracture
▸ Identified 676 patients treated with early fracture care.

Hak DJ.
Rapid Reference Review in Orthopedic Trauma:
Pivotal Papers Revealed (pp 289-295).
© 2013 SLACK Incorporated.

- Compared them to 906 patients from the American College of Surgeons Multiple Trauma Outcomes Study data (assumed that these patients did not undergo early fracture care).

Results

- Mortality was significantly reduced in the patients who had early total care of all their injuries including fracture stabilization.
- Subgroup of patients < 50 years of age
  - ▷ ISS of 18 to 34
    - » Mortality reduction from 11.8% to 5.1% with early fracture care (*P* < .01)
  - ▷ ISS 35 to 45
    - » Mortality reduction from 25.8% to 11.5% (*P* < .01) with early fracture care
- Subgroup of patients > 50 years of age
  - ▷ ISS 18 to 34
    - » Mortality reduction from 26.4% to 8% with early fracture care (*P* < .01)
  - ▷ ISS 35 to 45
    - » Mortality reduction from 42.3% to 18.4% with early fracture care (*P* < .05)

Conclusions

- The authors concluded that this study clearly shows the additional benefit of early fracture stabilization in reducing mortality rates in the patient with multiple injuries.

Commentary

- During the decade prior to this publication, several studies began to show the benefit of early skeletal stabilization in multiply injured patients (see Bone et al, [*J Bone Joint Surg Am*. 1989;71:336–340] in Chapter 11).
- The thinking prior to these studies, and the current study, was that multiply injured patients were too sick to undergo fracture stabilization.
- These papers changed the treatment paradigm from too sick to undergo early fracture stabilization to too sick not to undergo early fracture stabilization.

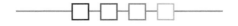

FEATURED ARTICLE

Authors: Pape HC, Auf'm'Kolk M, Paffrath T, Regel G, Sturm JA, Tscherne H.

Title: Primary intramedullary femur fixation in multiple trauma patients with associated lung contusion—a cause of posttraumatic ARDS?

Journal Information: *J Trauma*. 1993;34(4):540–547;discussion 547–548.

Study Design: Retrospective Review

- 106 multiply injured patients with femoral shaft fractures.
- Inclusion criteria
  - ISS > 18
  - Midshaft femur fracture treated with IM nail
  - Primary admission or referral within 8 hours after injury
  - No death from head injury or hemorrhagic shock
- 2 groups were differentiated according to the presence or absence of chest trauma.
- These 2 groups were then differentiated according to the time of femur stabilization
  - Severe chest trauma = Abbreviated Injury Scale (AIS) thorax ≥ 2
    - IM nail < 24 hours after injury (24 patients)
    - IM nail > 24 hours after injury (26 patients)
  - No severe chest trauma = AIS thorax < 2
    - IM nail < 24 hours after injury (33 patients)
    - IM nail > 24 hours after injury (23 patients)

Results

- ISS
  - Severe chest trauma and IM nail < 24 hours: 29.4
  - Severe chest trauma and IM nail > 24 hours: 31.4
  - No chest trauma and IM nail < 24 hours: 20.1
  - No chest trauma and IM nail > 24 hours: 25.4

- In the absence of severe chest trauma, the intensive care unit (ICU) time and intubation time were lower in patients treated with primary (< 24 hours from injury) IM nailing
  - ▷ Average time in ICU
    - » 7.3 days in group with no chest trauma and IM nail < 24 hours
    - » 18 days in group with no chest trauma and IM nail > 24 hours
  - ▷ Average intubation time
    - » 5.5 days in group with no chest trauma and IM nail < 24 hours
    - » 11 days in group with no chest trauma and IM nail > 24 hours
- In patients with severe chest trauma, there was a higher incidence of post-traumatic acute respiratory distress syndrome (ARDS) and mortality when early IM femoral nailing was done
  - ▷ ARDS
    - » 33% in group with severe chest trauma and IM nail < 24 hours
    - » 7.7% in group with severe chest trauma and IM nail > 24 hours
  - ▷ Mortality
    - » 21% in group with severe chest trauma and IM nail < 24 hours
    - » 4% in group with severe chest trauma and IM nail > 24 hours

Conclusions

- In the absence of severe chest trauma, primary (< 24 hours from injury) IM femoral nailing is beneficial.
- In the presence of severe chest trauma, primary (< 24 hours from injury) IM femoral nailing is associated with a higher incidence of ARDS and mortality.

Commentary

- This article initiated a swing in the pendulum from early total fracture care in multiply injured patients.
- The authors have suggested that there may be a subgroup of multiply injured patients, specifically those with severe chest trauma, in whom early fracture stabilization with an IM nail may be detrimental.

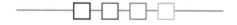

FEATURED ARTICLE
Authors: Pape HC, Grimme K, Van Griensven M, et al.

Title: Impact of intramedullary instrumentation versus damage control for femoral fractures on immunoinflammatory parameters: prospective randomized analysis by the EPOFF Study Group.

Journal Information: *J Trauma.* 2003;55(1):7–13.

Study Design: Prospective, Randomized, Multicenter Intervention Study

▸ Designed to study the effects of different types of fracture stabilization on the systemic release of proinflammatory cytokines in clinically stable patients with multiple injuries.

▸ Inclusion criteria

  ▷ Lower extremity long bone shaft fracture

  ▷ ISS > 16 or more than 3 extremity injuries (AIS score of ≥ 2) in association with another injury

  ▷ Thoracic AIS score < 4

  ▷ Age 18 to 65 years

▸ Randomization (computer generated) for the treatment of long bone fracture was performed at admission

  ▷ 17 patients—primary IM nail within 24 hours of injury

  ▷ 18 patients—damage control orthopedics (DCO) group initially treated with external fixation

▸ Serially sampled central venous blood was assessed for

  ▷ IL-1

  ▷ IL-6

  ▷ IL-8

▸ Timing of sample draws

  ▷ At the end of emergency room treatment

  ▷ Intraoperatively at 30 minutes after skin incision

▷ Postop 7 hours after skin incision

▷ Postop 24 hours after skin incision

▷ In the DCO group, samples were again taken at the time of conversion to IM nail

▸ Evaluated clinical parameters and complications (acute respiratory distress syndrome, multiple organ failure, sepsis).

Results

▸ No differences in complication rates (acute respiratory distress syndrome, sepsis, or multiple organ failure) between the 2 treatment groups.

▸ Systemic levels of IL-1 did not change during the perioperative period, and there was no difference in systemic levels of IL-1 levels between the 2 groups.

▸ Systemic IL-6 levels increased significantly from preop to postop in the primary IM nail group (P = .03) but not in the DCO group

  ▷ Primary IM nail group

    ≫ Preop: 55 ± 33 pg/dL

    ≫ 24 hours postop: 254 ± 55 pg/dL

  ▷ DCO group at time of initial external fixation

    ≫ Preop: 71 ± 42 pg/dL

    ≫ 24 hours postop: 68 ± 34 pg/dL

  ▷ DCO group at time of delayed conversion to IM nail

    ≫ Preop: 36 ± 21 pg/dL

    ≫ 24 hours postop: 39 ± 25 pg/dL

▸ Similarly, significant increases were seen in IL-8 levels in primary IM nail group between preop and 7 hours postop levels (P < .05), but not in the DCO group

  ▷ Primary IM nail group

    ≫ Preop: 35 ± 29 pg/dL

    ≫ 7 hours postop: 95 ± 23 pg/dL

  ▷ DCO group at time of initial external fixation

    ≫ Preop: 43 ± 38 pg/dL

    ≫ 24 hours postop: 69 ± 39 pg/dL

  ▷ DCO group at time of delayed conversion to IM nail

    ≫ Preop: 25 ± 20 pg/dL

    ≫ 24 hours postop: 36 ± 29 pg/dL

Conclusions

▶ A sustained inflammatory response was measured after primary (<24 hours after injury) IM nailing but not after initial external fixation or after secondary conversion to an IM nail.

▶ These findings may become clinically relevant in patients at high risk of developing complications.

▶ This study confirms previous studies that damage control orthopedic surgery appears to minimize the additional surgical impact induced by acute IM femoral nailing.

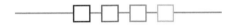

REVIEW ARTICLES

Flierl MA, Stoneback JW, Beauchamp KM, et al. Femur shaft fracture fixation in head-injured patients: when is the right time? *J Orthop Trauma.* 2010;24(2):107–114.

Pape HC, Tornetta P III, Tarkin I, Tzioupis C, Sabeson V, Olson SA. Timing of fracture fixation in multitrauma patients: the role of early total care and damage control surgery. *J Am Acad Orthop Surg.* 2009;17(9):541–549.

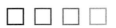

Open Fractures

chapter **30**

CLASSIC ARTICLE

Authors: Gustilo RB, Anderson JT.

Title: Prevention of infection in the treatment of one thousand and twenty-five open fractures of long bones: retrospective and prospective analyses.

Journal Information: *J Bone Joint Surg Am.* 1976;58(4):453–458.

Study Design: Includes Both a Retrospective Review and a Prospective Study

▶ Defines the commonly used Gustilo-Anderson classification of open fractures

  ▷ Type I: wound less than 1 cm long and clean

  ▷ Type II: laceration more than 1 cm long without extensive soft-tissue damage, flaps, or avulsions

  ▷ Type III: either an open segmental fracture, an open fracture with extensive soft-tissue damage, or a traumatic amputation

   » Special categories of injuries that were defined as type III also included gunshot injuries, any open fracture caused by a farm injury, and any open fracture with vascular injury requiring repair

Hak DJ.
Rapid Reference Review in Orthopedic Trauma: Pivotal Papers Revealed (pp 297-308).
© 2013 SLACK Incorporated.

- ▸ Retrospective review of 673 open long bone fractures (tibia and fibula, femur, radius and ulna, humerus) treated from 1955 to 1968
  - ▷ 1955 to 1960 infection rate was 12%
  - ▷ 1961 to 1968 infection rate was 5%
- ▸ Prospective study of open fractures managed with a standard protocol from 1969 to 1973
  - ▷ 352 open long bone fractures treated
  - ▷ 326 of these had a minimum 6 weeks follow-up
  - ▷ All treated with a protocol that included
    - » Débridement and copious irrigation (average of 10 to 14 L normal saline)
    - » Primary closure of type I and II fractures
    - » Secondary closure for type III fractures
    - » No primary internal fixation except in the presence of associated vascular injuries
    - » Culture of all wounds
    - » Antibiotics (oxacillin-ampicillin) before surgery and for 3 days postop
  - ▷ 158 of these open wounds had complete culture results
  - ▷ 70% (111/158) had a contaminated wound as shown by a positive wound culture
    - » 80 had a positive wound culture on admission
    - » 31 additional patients had a positive culture following débridement
  - ▷ 86 isolates of bacteria were gram-positive
  - ▷ 47 isolates of bacteria were gram-negative
  - ▷ Based on the sensitivities of these organisms, cephalosporins were found to be the most effective antibiotics for open-fracture prophylaxis
  - ▷ 8 (2.4%) of the 326 fractures in the prospective study became infected compared to 24 (5.2%) of the 548 open fractures treated in the 8-year period prior to institution of the open-fracture treatment protocol
  - ▷ The 9.9% infection rate in type III fractures was significantly lower than the 44% seen in type III fractures in the retrospective study group ($P < .01$)

Conclusions

- ▸ Open fractures require emergency treatment, including adequate débridement and copious irrigation.

- Primary closure is indicated for type I and II open fractures, but delayed primary closure, including split-thickness skin grafts or appropriate flaps, should be used for type III open fractures.
- Internal fixation by plates or IM nails should not be used. External skeletal fixation by skeletal traction, pins incorporated in a plaster cast, or external fixation is recommended.
- Open fractures associated with arterial injury requiring repair should be treated in skeletal traction whenever possible instead of by primary internal fixation.
- Antibiotics should be administered before and during surgery, the antibiotics of choice currently being cephalosporins. If the wound is closed primarily, antibiotics are stopped on the third postop day. If the wound is closed secondarily, the antibiotics are continued for another 3 days.

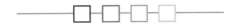

FEATURED ARTICLE

Authors: Gustilo RB, Mendoza RM, Williams DN.

Title: Problems in the management of type III (severe) open fractures: a new classification of type III open fractures.

Journal Information: *J Trauma.* 1984;24(8):742–746.

Study Design: Retrospective Review

- Defined subclassifications for type III open fractures.
- The authors indicated that, because of the varied severity and prognosis, their prior designation of type III open fracture is too inclusive, and therefore recommended that they be divided into 3 subtypes in order of worsening prognosis
    1. Type IIIA: adequate soft-tissue coverage of a fractured bone despite extensive soft-tissue laceration or flaps, or high-energy trauma irrespective of the size of the wound
    2. Type IIIB: extensive soft-tissue injury loss with periosteal stripping and bone exposure
    3. Type IIIC: open fracture associated with arterial injury requiring repair

▸ Retrospective review of 87 type III open fractures (in 75 patients) treated from 1976 to 1979.

Results

▸ Wound infection rates
  ▷ Type IIIA: 4%
  ▷ Type IIIB: 52%
  ▷ Type IIIC: 42%
▸ Amputation rates
  ▷ Type IIIA: 0%
  ▷ Type IIIB: 16%
  ▷ Type IIIC: 42%
▸ Factors leading to increased morbidity in type III fractures were
  ▷ Massive soft-tissue damage
  ▷ Compromised vascularity
  ▷ Severe wound contamination
  ▷ Marked fracture instability

Conclusions

▸ The authors noted that the bacterial pathogens in infected open fractures changed dramatically over the years
  ▷ In this series (1976 to 1979), 77% of wounds were contaminated with gram-negative bacteria
  ▷ In their prior series (1961 to 1975), only 24% had gram-negative bacteria
  ▷ Recommended a change of antibiotic therapy for type III open fractures from a first-generation cephalosporin alone to a combination of a cephalosporin and an aminoglycoside or a third-generation cephalosporin

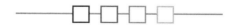

FEATURED ARTICLE

Authors: Petrisor B, Sun X, Bhandari M, et al.

Title: Fluid lavage of open wounds (FLOW): a multicenter, blinded, factorial pilot trial comparing alternative irrigating solutions and pressures in patients with open fractures.

Journal Information: *J Trauma.* 2011;71(3):596–606.

Study Design: Prospective, Randomized 2 × 2 Factorial (Patients Randomized Into 1 of 4 Groups), Multicenter (9 Sites in Canada and United States), Pilot Trial of 111 Patients With Open Fractures

▸ Randomized to treatment with either of the following:
  ▷ Castile soap solution or normal saline
  ▷ High- or low-pressure pulsatile lavage
▸ Primary outcome
  ▷ All unplanned reoperations (for infection, wound healing problems, and nonunions) within 1 year of the initial operative procedure
▸ Secondary outcomes
  ▷ Infections
  ▷ Wound healing problems
  ▷ Nonunions
  ▷ Functional outcomes scores
    » Euro quality of life-5 dimensions (EQ-5D)
    » SF-12
▸ 89 patients completed 1-year follow-up.

Results

▸ Primary outcome events in the castile soap and saline groups were not significantly different (hazard ratio: 0.91; 95% confidence interval: 0.42 to 2.00; P = .52)

 ▷ 13 (23%) in the castile soap group

 ▷ 13 (24%) in the saline group

▸ Primary outcome events in high- and low-pressure groups were not significantly different (hazard ratio: 0.55; 95% confidence interval [CI]: 0.24 to 1.27; P = .17)

 ▷ 16 (28%) in the high-pressure group

 ▷ 10 (19%) in the low-pressure group

▸ No significant difference between groups in functional outcome scores at any time point.

Conclusions

▸ This pilot study demonstrated the possibility that the use of low pressure may decrease the reoperation rate for infection, wound healing problems, or nonunion.

▸ The results of this pilot study have led the investigators to perform a larger-scale study to further evaluate this possibility.

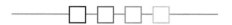

FEATURED ARTICLE
Author: Anglen JO.
Title: Comparison of soap and antibiotic solutions for irrigation of lower-limb open fracture wounds. A prospective, randomized study.
Journal Information: *J Bone Joint Surg Am.* 2005;87(7): 1415–1422.

Study Design: Prospective, Randomized Study (by Drawing a Card From an Envelope)

- 400 adult patients with 458 open fractures enrolled over 7.75 years
  - ▷ 192 patients received bacitracin solution
  - ▷ 208 patients received castile soap solution
- 49 patients with 55 open fractures were lost to follow-up.
- 351 patients with 403 open fractures comprised the study group
  - ▷ 171 patients with 199 open fractures in bacitracin group
  - ▷ 180 patients with 199 open fractures in castile soap group
- Randomized to open fracture irrigation with
  - ▷ Bacitracin solution (100,000 u/3 L normal saline)
  - ▷ Castile soap solution (80 mL/3 L normal saline)
  - ▷ Solution delivered in normal saline with a Pulsavac power irrigator (Zimmer, Warsaw, IN)
    - » 3 L for type I open fractures
    - » 6 L for type II open fractures
    - » 9 L for type III open fractures
  - ▷ Number of planned débridements per protocol
    - » 1 débridement for type I open
    - » 2 débridements for type II open
    - » 3 débridements for type III open
    - » However, there was frequent deviation from the protocol
  - ▷ Wound cultures were obtained before and after each débridement
- Primary outcome measures
  - ▷ Wound infection (superficial and deep)
  - ▷ Nonunion or delayed union
  - ▷ Failure of soft-tissue healing
- Patients were followed until they developed an infectious or healing complication or until they were discharged from care with a healed fracture and healed soft tissues.
- Average follow-up of all patients: 500 days (35 to 2422 days).
- Minimum follow-up prior to discharge of patients with a healed fracture and no wound complications was 180 days.
- No difference between the bacitracin and castile soap groups in terms of the following:
  - ▷ Gender
  - ▷ Gustilo-Anderson grade of the open fracture

▷ Time between injury and the irrigation

▷ Smoking

▷ Alcohol use

▸ Significant differences between the bacitracin and castile soap groups in terms of the following:

▷ Average age (38 in bacitracin group compared with 42, *P* = .01)

▷ Follow-up duration (560 days in bacitracin group compared with 444, *P* = .01)

▷ Hypotension (23% in bacitracin group compared with 14%, *P* = .04)

▷ Duration of IV antibiotics (11 days in bacitracin group compared with 9, *P* = .02)

Results

▸ Infection rate not significantly different (*P* = .2)

▷ 35/199 (18%) of fracture sites in bacitracin group

▷ 26/199 (18%) of fracture sites in castile soap group

▸ Delayed union rate not significantly different (*P* = .72)

▷ 49/199 (25%) delayed unions in bacitracin group

▷ 46/199 (23%) delayed unions in castile soap group

▸ Wound healing problem rate was significantly different (*P* = .03)

▷ 19/199 (9.5%) wound healing problems in bacitracin group

▷ 8/199 (4%) wound healing problems in castile soap group

Conclusions

▸ Irrigation of open fracture wounds with antibiotic solution offers no advantages over the use of a nonsterile soap solution.

▸ Irrigation of open fracture wounds with antibiotic solution may increase the risk of wound healing problems.

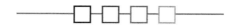

FEATURED ARTICLE

Authors: Stannard JP, Volgas DA, Stewart R, McGwin G Jr, Alonso JE.

Title: Negative pressure wound therapy after severe open fractures: a prospective randomized study.

Journal Information: *J Orthop Trauma.* 2009;23(8):552–557.

Study Design: Prospective, Randomized Study (Using a Random Sampling Algorithm in a 1:1 Ratio)

- ▸ 62 severe high-energy open fractures.
- ▸ Inclusion criteria to define severe high-energy open fractures
  - ▷ Heavily contaminated type II fractures
  - ▷ Type IIIA fractures that were heavily contaminated or had severe soft-tissue injury
  - ▷ All type IIIB and type IIIC fractures
- ▸ All treated with irrigation and débridement, which was repeated every 48 to 72 hours until the wound was closed.
- ▸ Randomized to wound treatment with the following:
  - ▷ Fine mesh gauze—25 fractures in 23 patients
  - ▷ Negative pressure wound therapy (Wound VAC, Kinetic Concepts, Inc, San Antonio, TX)—37 fractures in 35 patients
- ▸ Average follow-up: 28 months (14 to 67 months).
- ▸ Average number of repeat débridements prior to wound closure/coverage
  - ▷ 2.4 in control group
  - ▷ 2.7 in Wound VAC group
- ▸ Primary outcome measurements
  - ▷ Deep wound infection/osteomyelitis

Results

- ▸ Significantly fewer total infections in the Wound VAC group (P = .024)
  - ▷ Total infections
    - » 28% (7/25) in control group
    - » 5.4% (2/35) in Wound VAC group
  - ▷ Acute infections
    - » 8% (2/25) in control group
    - » 0% in Wound VAC group
  - ▷ Delayed infections
    - » 20% (5/25) in control group
    - » 5.4% (2/35) in Wound VAC group
- ▸ Relative risk ratio is 0.199, suggesting that patients treated with a Wound VAC were one-fifth as likely to develop an infection of their open fracture.

Conclusions

▶ The authors suggest that the Wound VAC is an effective adjunct along with surgical débridement and IV antibiotics in the treatment of severe open fractures.

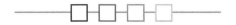

FEATURED ARTICLE
Authors: Lenarz CJ, Watson JT, Moed BR, Israel H, Mullen JD, Macdonald JB.
Title: Timing of wound closure in open fractures based on cultures obtained after debridement.
Journal Information: *J Bone Joint Surg Am.* 2010;92(10): 1921–1926.

Study Design: Retrospective Review

▶ 422 open fractures treated between March 2003 and December 2005 using a standard protocol that used wound cultures as a guide for timing of wound closure.

▶ 346 cases were available for long-term follow-up (duration not specifically defined).

▶ Protocol

▷ Wound cultures (aerobic and anaerobic) were obtained following débridement

▷ At 48 hours after débridement, patients returned to surgery

» If initial cultures were negative, the wound was closed

» If initial cultures were positive, a repeat irrigation and débridement was performed, and additional cultures were obtained after débridement

» Serial débridement was repeated, and the wound was not closed until cultures were negative

▷ Wounds were irrigated with pulsatile lavage

» Type I open fractures with 3 L normal saline

» Type II open fractures with 6 L normal saline

» Type III open fractures with 9 L normal saline

▸ Average age: 38 years (15 to 92 years), 249 males, 97 females.

▸ 12 patients had multiple open fractures, and each fracture was evaluated individually.

▸ Fracture classification

  ▷ 50 type I open

  ▷ 123 type II open

  ▷ 111 type IIIA open

  ▷ 47 type IIIB open

  ▷ 15 type IIIC open (9 underwent amputation)

▸ Variations from protocol

  ▷ Decision to close type I fractures primarily was at surgeon's discretion

  ▷ 73 patients with low-energy injuries and negative wound cultures were not returned to the operating room, and their wounds were allowed to heal by secondary intention

  ▷ While most type II and type III wounds were left open, 32 selected type II wounds were loosely closed following the initial débridement

Results

▸ Overall deep infection rate: 4.3%.

▸ Type I deep infection rate: 0%.

▸ Type II deep infection rate: 4% (5/123).

▸ Type III deep infection: 5.7% (10/173)

  ▷ Type IIIA deep infection rate: 1.8% (2/111)

  ▷ Type IIB deep infection rate: 10.6% (5/47)

  ▷ Type IIIC deep infection rate: 20% (3/15)

  ▷ There was a significant difference in the 3 type III categories ($P = .003$)

▸ Average: 2.6 débridements per fracture.

▸ Fractures in which the wound was closed despite positive cultures (a protocol breach) did not have a significantly increased risk of deep infection ($P = .0501$).

- ▶ Higher infection rates found in the following:
  - ▷ Fractures requiring multiple débridements (P = .002)
    - ≫ Average: 3.8 débridements in patients developing deep infection
    - ≫ Average: 2.5 débridements in fractures that did not develop infection
  - ▷ Fractures in patients with diabetes
    - ≫ Relative risk: 4.2 (P = .043)
  - ▷ Fractures in patients with an increased body mass index (P = .047)
    - ≫ 1.6% in patients with body mass index (BMI) < 25 kg/m²
    - ≫ 6% in patients with BMI ≥ 25 kg/m²
- ▶ No difference seen in infection rates in upper versus lower extremity fractures.

Conclusions

- ▶ Use of this standardized protocol was shown to achieve a very low rate of deep infection compared with historical controls (prior publication rates have ranged from 7% to 22%).
- ▶ An increased number of irrigation and débridement procedures is required to achieve this lowered rate of deep infection.

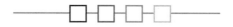

REVIEW ARTICLES
Weitz-Marshall AD, Bosse MJ. Timing of closure of open fractures. *J Am Acad Orthop Surg.* 2002;10(6):379–384.
Zalavras CG, Patzakis, MJ. Open fractures: evaluation and management. *J Am Acad Orthop Surg.* 2003;11(3):212–219.

Periprosthetic Fractures

chapter **31**

FEATURED ARTICLE

Authors: Ricci WM, Bolhofner BR, Loftus T, Cox C, Mitchell S, Borrelli J Jr.

Title: Indirect reduction and plate fixation, without grafting, for periprosthetic femoral shaft fractures about a stable intramedullary implant.

Journal Information: *J Bone Joint Surg Am* 2005;87(10): 2240–2245.

Study Design: Prospective Consecutive Case Series

▶ 50 patients with a periprosthetic femur fracture distal to a stable hip arthroplasty (Vancouver type-B1 fracture).

▶ All treated with minimally invasive approach, indirect reduction, extraperiosteal lateral plate fixation without bone graft or strut grafts.

▶ Proximal fixation with a combination of standard screws and cables.

▶ Distal fixation with screws.

▶ Follow-up

  ▷ 4 patients died

  ▷ 5 patients had inadequate follow-up

  ▷ 41 patients were followed an average: 24 months (11 to 170 months)

▶ Average age: 72 years (38 to 98 years), 15 males, 26 females.

Hak DJ.
*Rapid Reference Review in Orthopedic Trauma:
Pivotal Papers Revealed (pp 309-313).*
© 2013 SLACK Incorporated.

Results

- ▸ All fractures healed.
- ▸ Average time to union: 12 weeks (7 to 23 weeks).
- ▸ Average time to weightbearing as tolerated: 12 weeks (7 to 32 weeks).
- ▸ Complications
  - ▷ 1 deep infection
  - ▷ 3 hardware failures
    - » 1 patient fractured 1 cable
    - » 2 patients fractured 1 screw
    - » All 3 healed without evidence of implant loosening or malalignment
- ▸ 30 patients returned to their baseline ambulatory status.
- ▸ 11 patients had either a decline in their ambulatory status and/or a need for additional assistive devices at their last follow-up.

Conclusions

- ▸ This study supports the use of indirect reduction and internal fixation with a single extraperiosteal plate, without the use of allograft struts, for the treatment of periprosthetic fractures about a stable hip arthroplasty.

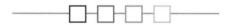

FEATURED ARTICLE

Authors: Ricci WM, Loftus T, Cox C, Borrelli J.

Title: Locked plates combined with minimally invasive insertion technique for the treatment of periprosthetic supracondylar femur fractures above a total knee arthroplasty.

Journal Information: *J Orthop Trauma.* 2006;20(3):190–196.

Study Design: Prospective Consecutive Case Series

▸ 24 supracondylar femur fractures above a well-fixed nonstemmed total knee arthroplasty in 22 patients.

▸ All treated with indirect reduction, locking condylar plating, and no bone graft.

▸ 1 patient died, and 1 was lost to follow-up.

▸ Average follow-up: 15 months (6 to 45 months).

▸ Average age: 70 years (50 to 95 years), 5 males, 15 females.

▸ Outcome measurements

  ▷ Ambulatory status

  ▷ Radiographic evaluation

    » Fracture alignment

    » Fracture healing

Results

▸ 86% (19/22 fractures) union rate.

▸ Average time to unrestricted weightbearing

  ▷ 12 weeks (8 to 20 weeks) for patients without fixation failure

  ▷ 14 weeks (10 to 18 weeks) for patients with fixation failure

▸ Ambulatory status

  ▷ 3 patients with healing complications became nonambulatory

  ▷ 15/17 patients who healed their fractures returned to their baseline ambulatory status

  ▷ 2/17 patient who healed their fractures changed from community ambulators to household ambulators

▸ Complications

  ▷ 3 nonunions

    » All 3 patients were insulin-dependent diabetics and obese

    » 2 infected nonunions

    » 1 aseptic nonunion

  ▷ 2 malalignments (> 5 degrees)

  ▷ 4 patients had fracture of proximal screws

    » 3 of these were associated with progressive coronal plane deformity

Conclusions

▶ The authors concluded that fixation of periprosthetic supracondylar femur fractures with a locking condylar plate provides satisfactory results in nondiabetic patients.

▶ The authors expressed caution regarding a high risk for healing complications and infections in diabetic patients.

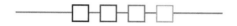

FEATURED ARTICLE

Authors: Gliatis J, Megas P, Panagiotopoulos E, Lambiris E.

Title: Midterm results of treatment with a retrograde nail for supracondylar periprosthetic fractures of the femur following total knee arthroplasty.

Journal Information: *J Orthop Trauma.* 2005;19(3):164–170.

Study Design: Cohort Study

▶ 10 periprosthetic femur fractures in 9 patients treated with retrograde supracondylar nail

  ▷ 1 occurred intraoperatively

  ▷ Average time from arthroplasty to fracture in other cases: 33 months (2 weeks to 7 years)

▶ Average age: 70 years (52 to 83 years), 1 male, 8 females.

▶ Average follow-up: 34.5 months (25 to 52 months).

▶ Outcome measurements

  ▷ Western Ontario and McMaster Universities Osteoarthritis Index (WOMAC)

  ▷ Radiographic evaluation

Results

- All fractures united within 3 months.
- 1 malunion (35 degrees valgus).
- No infections.
- No prosthetic loosening.
- Trend for lower WOMAC scores postop but not statistically significant.

Conclusions

- The authors concluded retrograde nailing is a reliable technique for treatment of periprosthetic supracondylar fractures with minimal morbidity and a low complication rate.

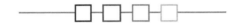

REVIEW ARTICLES

McGraw P, Kumar A. Periprosthetic fractures of the femur after total knee arthroplasty. *J Orthop Traumatol.* 2010;11(3):135–141.

Pike J, Davidson D, Garbuz D, Duncan CP, O'Brien PJ, Masri BA. Principles of treatment for periprosthetic femoral shaft fractures around well-fixed total hip arthroplasty. *J Am Acad Orthop Surg.* 2009;17(11):677–688.

Steinmann SP, Cheung EV. Treatment of periprosthetic humerus fractures associated with shoulder arthroplasty. *J Am Acad Orthop Surg.* 2008;16(4):199–207.

Su ET, DeWal H, Di Cesare PE. Periprosthetic femoral fractures above total knee replacements. *J Am Acad Orthop Surg.* 2004;12(1):12–20.